Handbook

of the Common

Acute Infectious Diseases

Illustrated in Full Color

Published Exclusively for the Medical Profession by

AURALGAN RESEARCH DIVISION

NEW YORK, N. Y., U. S. A.

Adapted from

CLINICAL PEDIATRICS

BY

I. NEWTON KUGELMASS, M.D., Ph.D., Sc.D.

ILLUSTRATED

BY

EVE MADSEN

• Contents •

PREFACE

THE pathognomonic signs of the Acute Infectious Diseases are familiar to clinicians but their association with less obvious sequelae are often forgotten. The illustrations of each infectious disease are arranged chronologically in terms of typical manifestations, clinical course and common sequelae. These visual features are correlated with a factual review of the basic principles of everyday problems in infectious diseases. A bibliography accompanies each disorder. This work will, it is hoped, provide adequate information on the acute infectious diseases in convenient compass.

CHICKENPOX

(VARICELLA)

NATURE

Varicella is characterized by an erythematous eruption of papules and vesicles involving the skin of the entire body and the mucous membranes of the mouth and throat, accompanied by mild constitutional symptoms.

ETIOLOGY

A filtrable virus is contained in the vesicles.
It may be transmitted by direct contact, fomites or a third person.
The greatest incidence is in fall and winter.
Infants under 6 months of age are relatively immune.
One attack confers permanent immunity.
The period of incubation is 15 days or as long as 21 days.

SYMPTOMS

A prodromal period is uncommon although a fine rash may occur.
The onset is abrupt with appearance of small red macules or papules.
The rash develops over the trunk, scalp, face and extremities in this sequence, accompanied by moderate fever.
Large, round tear-drop, umbilicated vesicles form in many but not all of the macules.
The lesions may become turbid or purulent and quite itchy.
The vesicles dry up with the formation of crusts which drop off within a week and leave scars if secondarily infected.
Lesions may be present on the mucous membranes of the mouth and throat.
Complications such as impetigo, cellulitis, erysipelas, glomerular nephritis, encephalitis are uncommon but do occur.

TREATMENT

Isolation in quarantine should be maintained for 10 days or until the crusts have disappeared.
Temporary immunity can be maintained by intramuscular injection of 20 cc. of convalescent serum.
Bed rest, restraint from scratching and sedatives prevent secondary infection.
Lesions covered with metaphen in collodion (1:500) cannot be scratched.
Warm soda baths or $KMnO_4$ (1:5000) dressings are helpful.
2% ammoniated mercury or 5% sulfathiazole ointment with 1% phenol may be applied to prevent impetigo when crusts have formed.

CLINICAL COURSE OF CHICKENPOX

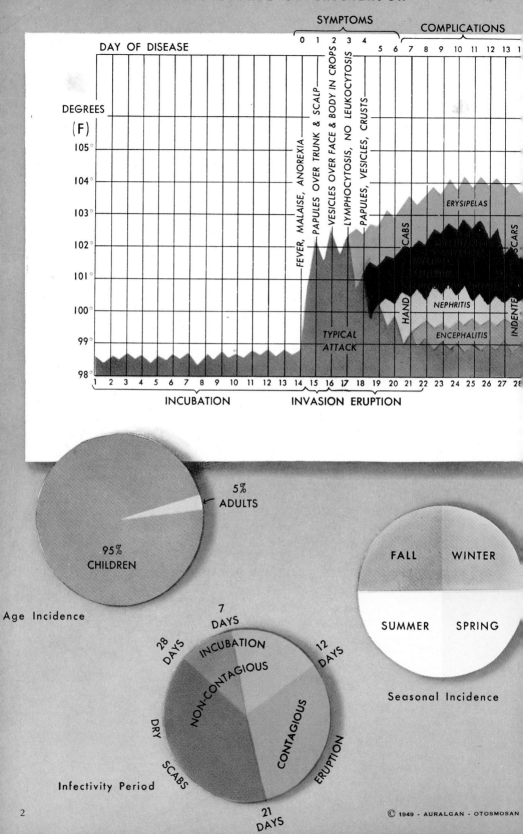

SYMPTOMS

COMPLICATIONS

DAY OF DISEASE

0 1 2 3 4 5 6 7 8 9 10 11 12 13 1

DEGREES
(F)

105°
104°
103°
102°
101°
100°
99°
98°

FEVER, MALAISE, ANOREXIA
PAPULES OVER TRUNK & SCALP
VESICLES OVER FACE & BODY IN CROPS
LYMPHOCYTOSIS, NO LEUKOCYTOSIS
PAPULES, VESICLES, CRUSTS

ERYSIPELAS

SCABS

HAND

NEPHRITIS

ENCEPHALITIS

SCARS

INDENTE

TYPICAL ATTACK

1 2 3 4 5 6 7 8 9 10 11 12 13 14 15 16 17 18 19 20 21 22 23 24 25 26 27 28

INCUBATION

INVASION ERUPTION

5%
ADULTS

95%
CHILDREN

Age Incidence

FALL | WINTER

SUMMER | SPRING

Seasonal Incidence

7 DAYS

28 DAYS

INCUBATION

12 DAYS

NON-CONTAGIOUS

DRY

SCABS

CONTAGIOUS

ERUPTION

21 DAYS

Infectivity Period

2

© 1949 - AURALGAN - OTOSMOSAN

TYPICAL ATTACK OF CHICKENPOX

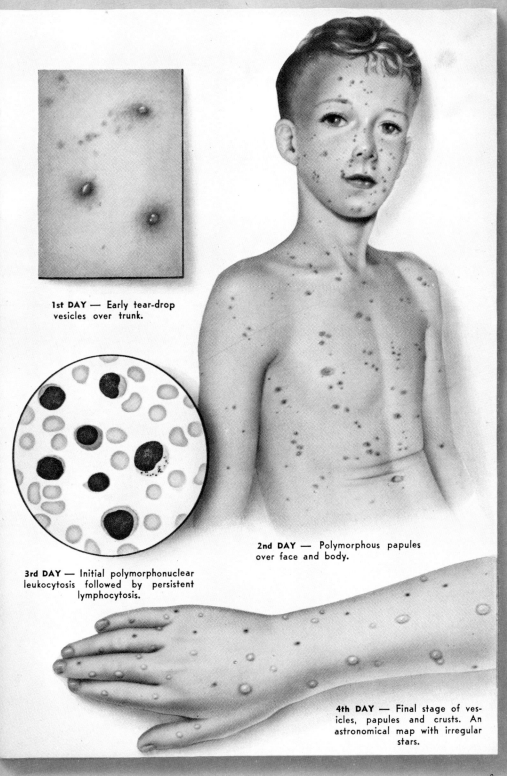

1st DAY — Early tear-drop vesicles over trunk.

3rd DAY — Initial polymorphonuclear leukocytosis followed by persistent lymphocytosis.

2nd DAY — Polymorphous papules over face and body.

4th DAY — Final stage of vesicles, papules and crusts. An astronomical map with irregular stars.

1949 · AURALGAN · OTOSMOSAN

COMPLICATIONS OF CHICKENPOX

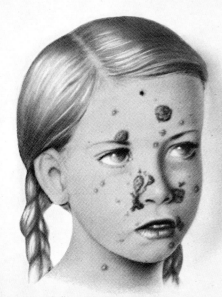

Bullous impetigo following
infected lesions.

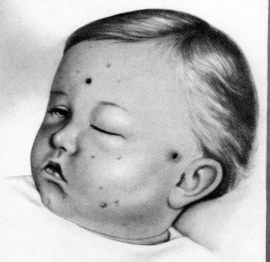

Cellulitis following infected lesions.

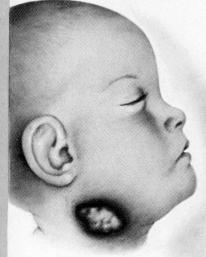

Suppurative Cervical Lymphadenitis
following severe attack.

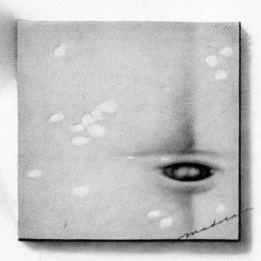

Scars years after an attack where scabs
were scratched and infected.

REFERENCES:

AMIES, C. R.: The Elementary Bodies of Varicella and Their Agglutination in Pure Suspension by the Serum of Chickenpox Patients, *Lancet, 1:*1015, 1933.

BLATT, M. L., ZELDERS, MARY, and STEIN, A. F.: Chickenpox Following Contact with Herpes Zoster, *J. Lab. and Clin. Med., 25:*951, 1940.

BRAIN, R. T.: The Relationship Between the Viruses of Zoster and Varicella as Demonstrated by the Complement-fixation Reaction, *Brit. J. Exper. Path., 14:* 67, 1933.

BULLOWA, J. G. M., and WISHIK, S. M.: Complications of Varicella, *Am. J. Dis. Child., 49:*923, 1935.

GORDON, J. E., and MEADER, F. M.: The Period of Infectivity and Serum Prevention of Chickenpox, *J.A.M.A., 93:*2013, 1929.

HABEL, K.: Mumps and Chickenpox as Air-Borne Diseases, *Am. J. M. Sc., 209:*75, 1945.

LAIDLAW, F. W.: Smallpox and Chickenpox—The Differential Diagnosis, *New York State J. Med., 28:*310, 1928.

LUCCHESI, P. F. *et al.*: Varicella Neonatorum, *Am. J. Dis. Child., 73:*44, 1947.

SHUMAN, H. H.: Varicella in the Newborn, *Am. J. Dis. Child., 58:*564, 1939.

WADDELL, W. W., JR., and ELEY, R. C.: Prophylaxis of Varicella with Vesicle Fluid, *Am. J. Dis. Child., 34:*540, 1927.

WESSELHOEFT, C.: The Differential Diagnosis of Chickenpox and Smallpox, *New England J. Med., 230:*15, 1944.

DIPHTHERIA

NATURE

This acute contagious disease is caused by Klebs-Loeffler bacillus. It is characterized by the formation of fibrinous exudate on the mucous membranes of the respiratory tract. Mild forms are without constitutional symptoms. Severe forms are attended by prostration, cardiac depression and severe anemia due to absorption of toxins. It is complicated by pneumonia and followed by localized or general paralysis.

ETIOLOGY

Transmitted by direct contact or by a carrier of virulent organisms. Spread by indirect contact with infected objects or unpasteurized and tainted milk. Communicability persists from virulent bacteria in nose and throat or other secretions. Organisms disappear in 2 to 4 weeks unless carrier state develops. Healthy carrier is a dangerous source of contagion. Children between 1 and 10 years, especially between 2 and 5 years, are mainly affected. Any infection of the nose and throat predisposes to diphtheria. Natural antitoxin or cellular immunity during the first 6 months of life occurs chiefly in temperate zones in the fall or winter. Epidemics have diminished since employment of active immunization.

SYMPTOMS

Incubation period is 2 to 5 days. Onset is preceded by fever, headache, malaise and sore throat. Symptoms are produced by toxins of the germ. Constitutional disturbances increase steadily with extension of the membrane formed over the upper respiratory tract.

TYPES

FAUCIAL

Onset is insidious. Pharynx is congested. Grayish exudate of membranous character appears on uvula, palate and pharyngeal wall. Membrane is quite adherent and sharply defined. Characteristic foul odor is present. Edema of pharynx develops. Cervical lymph nodes enlarge. Voice becomes husky, respiration noisy, swallowing difficult. Prostration is marked. Hemorrhages from the nose and throat occur occasionally. Albuminuria and hematuria are frequent at the onset.

NASAL

Occurs alone or associated with faucial infection. If limited to the nose, disease is mild. If nose and pharynx are involved, disease is malignant. Yellowish, bloodstained discharge appears from the nostrils. Membrane forms on inner or outer walls or posteriorly. Upper lip becomes excoriated.

CLINICAL COURSE OF DIPHTHERIA

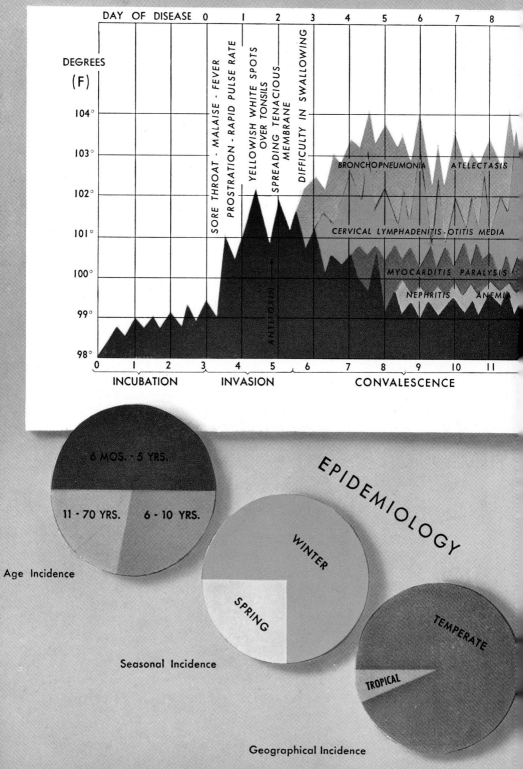

DAY OF DISEASE   0   1   2   3   4   5   6   7   8

DEGREES (F)

SORE THROAT - MALAISE - FEVER
PROSTRATION - RAPID PULSE RATE
YELLOWISH WHITE SPOTS OVER TONSILS
SPREADING TENACIOUS MEMBRANE
DIFFICULTY IN SWALLOWING

104°
103°
102°
101°
100°
99°
98°

ANTITOXIN

BRONCHOPNEUMONIA   ATELECTASIS
CERVICAL LYMPHADENITIS - OTITIS MEDIA
MYOCARDITIS PARALYSIS
NEPHRITIS   ANEMIA

0   1   2   3   4   5   6   7   8   9   10   11

INCUBATION   INVASION   CONVALESCENCE

6 MOS. - 5 YRS.

11 - 70 YRS.   6 - 10 YRS.

Age Incidence

EPIDEMIOLOGY

WINTER

SPRING

Seasonal Incidence

TEMPERATE

TROPICAL

Geographical Incidence

8

Mouth breathing is obvious. Nasal voice is common. Foreign body may simulate nasal diphtheria but it may arise with foreign body.

PHARYNGEAL
Primary or secondary to faucial form. Mechanical obstruction of glottis leads to cough, hoarseness, stridor, dyspnea and finally cyanosis. Without relief, death follows.

ATYPICAL
Membrane may occur in unusual regions—buccal cavity, lips, face, scalp, esophagus, stomach and intestinal tract. Membrane rarely occurs on conjunctiva, middle ear, skin, genitalia or unhealed umbilicus.

COMPLICATIONS

BRONCHOPNEUMONIA
Follows laryngeal involvement and severe sepsis, especially in infants.

HEART FAILURE
Most frequent between 5 and 12 days, following late antitoxin administration. May be abrupt causing sudden death after exertion.

NEPHRITIS
Urine contains albumin, casts, but rarely blood. Edema develops during second week. Renal insufficiency is rare. Recovery is usually rapid.

PARALYSIS
Peripheral neuritis may occur from second to fourth week. Paralysis of palate causes nasal speech and regurgitation of fluids. Other motor paralyses may involve ocular nerves, face, larynx, neck, arms or legs. Paralysis disappears after days or weeks. Diaphragmatic type is most fatal.

DIAGNOSIS

Immediate examination of a smear from the throat may reveal Klebs-Loeffler bacilli. Culture of membrane obtained by swab is more diagnostic. Negative results may occur in laryngeal diphtheria in absence of pharyngeal membrane. Single negative culture is inconclusive. Antitoxin administration depends on clinical rather than on bacterial criteria.

COURSE

Mild cases recover in a day or two. Usual course is a week of active symptoms followed by gradual recovery or death. Antitoxin results in improvement in 36 hours and recovery within a week. The younger the child the higher the mortality. Average mortality is 5% for all types.

PROPHYLAXIS

ACTIVE IMMUNITY
Infants between 6 months and 1 year of age should be immunized with toxoid. It is administered in 3 doses of 0.5, 1.0 and 1.5 cc. at 1 month in-

TYPICAL ATTACK OF DIPHTHERIA

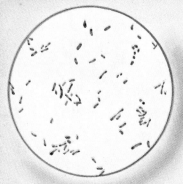

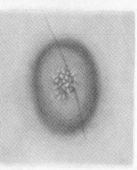

2nd DAY — Positive culture of diphtheria bacilli with clubbed ends and irregular stains.

3rd DAY — Positive Schick reactions in a child at 3 and 7 days respectively.

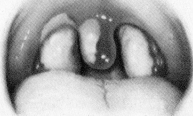

4th DAY — Grayish membrane spreading from tonsils to uvula over dusky red mucous membranes.

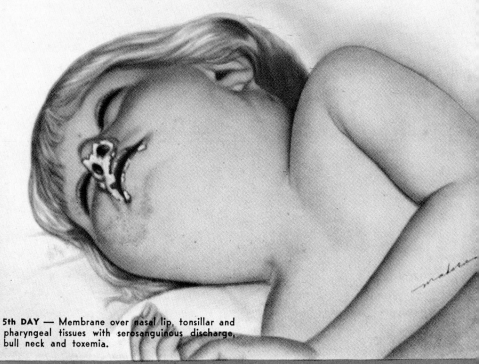

5th DAY — Membrane over nasal lip, tonsillar and pharyngeal tissues with serosanguinous discharge, bull neck and toxemia.

tervals. Schick test is performed 6 months later. If positive another series of injections is required. Immunity results after 2 months and lasts for 5 years.

PASSIVE IMMUNITY

Children exposed to diphtheria should have their immunity determined by Schick test. If positive, 1,000 units of antitoxin should be given. Serum confers immunity for 2 weeks.

SCHICK TEST

Inject intracutaneously on one forearm 0.1 cc. toxin solution containing 1/50 minimum lethal dose. Control of heated toxin is used on the opposite arm. Raised erythema in 24 to 48 hours over unaltered toxin means lack of immunity. Negative Schick and control tests indicate immunity.

TREATMENT

DIPHTHERIA ANTITOXIN

Infants should be given 5,000 units intramuscularly. Children require 8,000 units. Severe cases need up to 20,000 units intramuscularly or intravenously. Serum reactions are no cause for alarm.

SENSITIVITY TEST

History of allergy in the child or family is an indication for skin or conjunctival test. In nonallergic children 0.1 cc. of undiluted serum is injected intramuscularly. If a wheal does not appear within 20 minutes, proceed without hesitation. In allergic children make intradermal test with 0.05 cc. of 1:100 dilution or ophthalmic test with 1:100 dilution. If positive, desensitization by graduated doses is essential.

LARYNGEAL OBSTRUCTION

Remove membrane by suction or forceps. If edema causes suffocation, intubation tube must be inserted for one week or tracheotomy performed immediately.

LOCAL MEASURES

Irrigation is necessary to prevent aspiration of membrane into lungs. Gargles are helpful in older children. Procedure is contraindicated in nasal hemorrhage.

GENERAL MEASURES

Complete rest in bed is enforced for one month. Breast feeding is discontinued. Liquid diet is indicated. Gavage is essential in the presence of vomiting, difficult swallowing or nasal obstruction. Sedatives are necessary in laryngeal diphtheria or mild carditis. Cardiac stimulants are unnecessary. Intravenous dextrose solutions combat hypoglycemia.

SPECIFIC MEASURES

Secondary infection requires penicillin 20,000 I.U. q. 3 hrs. Myocarditis requires complete bed rest for one month. Insure massive vitamin B_1 and C

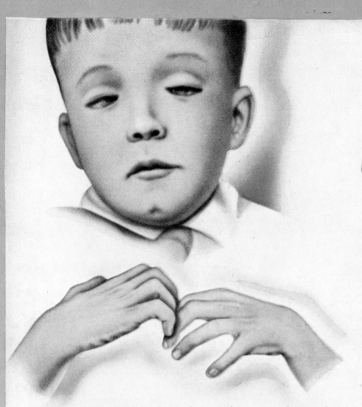

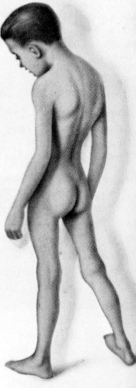

1 WEEK — Toxic neuritis with paralysis of the extra-ocular muscles causing strabismus and diplopia.

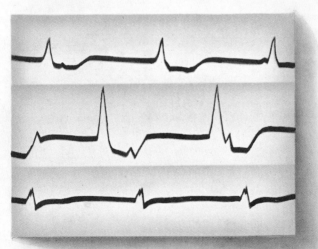

4 WEEKS — Progressive general paralysis of the face, neck, trunk and extremities with inability to raise the head and loss of sensation of position.

2 WEEKS — Toxic myocarditis with delay in conduction time and inversion of the T-wave in leads I and II.

intake. Give 70 cc. 50% dextrose intravenously q. 8 hrs. Paralysis of respiratory muscles requires Drinker respirator.

Paralysis of deglutition muscles is combated by keeping head low, decreasing salivation with atropin and feeding by gavage.

REFERENCES:

BRAHDY, M. B., LENARSKY, M., SMITH, L. W., and GAFFNEY, C. A.: A Rapid Method for the Identification of Diphtheria Bacilli, *J.A.M.A., 104*:1881, 1935.

BURKHARDT, E. A., EGGLESTON, CARY, and SMITH, L. W.: Electrocardiographic Changes and Peripheral Nerve Palsies in Toxic Diphtheria, *Am. J. M. Sc., 195*:301, 1938.

DOLGOLPOL, V. B., and MARKUS, H. V.: Rapid Diagnostic Method for Testing the Virulence of Corynebacteria, *J. Lab. and Clin. Med., 26*:553, 1940.

EDMUNDS, C. W.: Circulatory Collapse in Diphtheria, *Am. J. Dis. Child., 54*:1066, 1937.

FOX, W. W., RHOADS, P. S., and LACK, HERBERT: Experience with a Rapid Clinical Test for Diphtheria, *J.A.M.A., 113*:675, 1939.

FROBISHER, MARTIN, JR.: The Etiology of Malignant Diphtheria, *Am. J. Pub. Health, 33*:1244, 1943.

GORDON, J. E., YOUNG, D. D., and TOP, F. H.: Management by Mechanical Respirator of Postdiphtheritic Respiratory Paralysis, *J. Pediat., 3*:580, 1933.

JAREMA, J. J., and SMITH, L. W.: Relationship of the Morphology of the Diphtheria Bacillus to Its Virulence, *J. Infect. Dis., 55*:306, 1934.

KOCHER, R. A., and SIEMSEN, W. J.: Diphtheria Carriers Treated with Penicillin, *Ann. Int. Med., 24*:883, 1946.

MALONEY, P. J.: The Preparation and Testing of Diphtheria Toxoid, *Am. J. Pub. Health, 16*:1208, 1926.

NEFFSON, A. H., and WISHIK, S. M.: Acute Infectious Croup, *J. Pediat., 5*:433, 617 and 776, 1934.

PARK, W. H., and ZINGHER, A.: Active Immunization in Diphtheria and Treatment by Toxin-antitoxin, *J.A.M.A., 63*:859, 1914.

PERKINS, ROY F., and LAUFER, MAURICE W.: A Clinical Study of Post-diphtheritic Polyneuritis, *J. Nerv. and Ment. Dis., 104*:59, 1946.

POVITZKY, O. R., EISNER, M., and JACKSON, E.: Effectiveness of Standard Diphtheria Antitoxin Against All Types of Diphtheria Infections, *J. Infect. Dis., 52*:246, 1933.

RAMON, G., and HELIE, G. I.: Anatoxin as an Immunizing Agent Against Diphtheria, *Am. J. Dis. Child., 39*:685, 1930.

SCHWENTKER, F. F., and NOEL, W. W.: The Circulatory Failure of Diphtheria, *Bull. Johns Hopkins Hosp., 46*:359, 1930.

SELIGMANN, ERICH: Current Problems in Diphtheria, *New York State J. Med., 41*:136, 1941.

SMITH, THEOBALD: Active Immunity Produced by So-called Balanced or Neutral Mixtures of Diphtheria Toxin and Antitoxin, *J. Exper. Med., 11*:241, 1909.

SOLE, ALPHONS: Schnellkultur von Diphtheriebazillen, *Wein. klin. Wchnschr., 47*:713, 1934.

TOLLE, D. M.: Croup, *Am. J. Dis. Child., 39*:954, 1930.

TOOMEY, J. A.: Appraisals of Immunization Procedures, *Clinics, 2*:323, 1943.

WESSELHOEFT, CONRAD: Cardiovascular Disease in Diphtheria, *New England J. Med., 223*:57, 1940.

III

INFLUENZA

DEFINITION

Influenza means "under the influence," while grippe means "to attack."
Grippe is caused by a virus acting in association with other organisms.
It occurs pandemically, epidemically or endemically.
There is sudden onset with fever and prostration resulting from inflammation of the respiratory tract.
Severe nervous or gastro-intestinal manifestations invariably follow.
It is characterized by great explosiveness, high morbidity, high dispersiveness, low fatality.

ETIOLOGY

The primary incitant is influenza virus a, β or γ or another strain.
The Pfeiffer's bacillus or Hemophilus influenzae is a secondary invader.
It is associated with the specific virus attacking the upper respiratory tract.
Other organisms complicate influenza in pandemic and endemic types.
Epidemics usually occur in the late winter and early spring spread by air, droplet contamination and direct contact.
Epidemics occur in waves, the first being explosive and transient, while the others are more gradual and severe.
Communicability is possible as long as abnormal respiratory secretions persist.
Young children possess natural immunity and therefore escape the infection during serious epidemics.
Older children acquire transient immunity for several months.
Antibodies against the causative virus can be demonstrated during convalescence.
Similar antibodies have been found in the blood of contacts in subclinical cases.

TYPES

Pandemics are initiated by an unknown but virulent virus.
They are accompanied by bacterial infection of the respiratory tract.
Epidemics are initiated by viruses a, β or γ.
They are not accompanied by secondary invasion of the respiratory tract.
Endemics are initiated sporadically by an unknown virus.
They are always accompanied by a bacterial involvement of the respiratory tract.

CLINICAL COURSE OF INFLUENZA

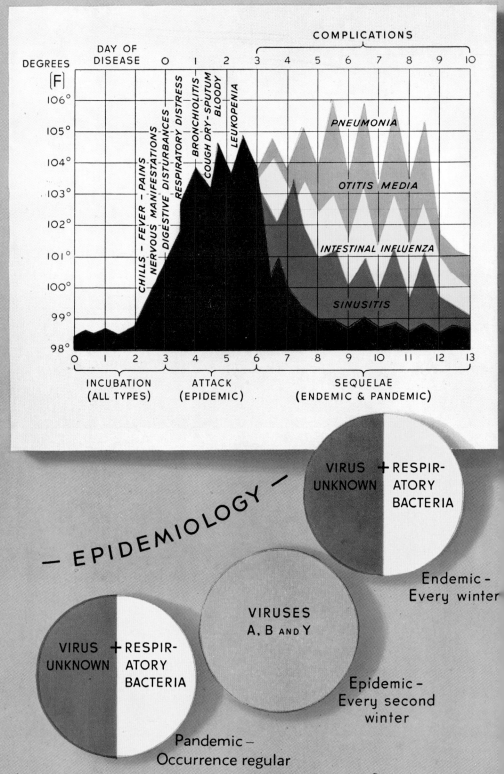

DEGREES
(F)

DAY OF DISEASE

COMPLICATIONS

0 1 2 3 4 5 6 7 8 9 10

106°
105°
104°
103°
102°
101°
100°
99°
98°

CHILLS – FEVER – PAINS
NERVOUS MANIFESTATIONS
DIGESTIVE DISTURBANCES
RESPIRATORY DISTRESS
BRONCHIOLITIS
COUGH DRY-SPUTUM BLOODY
LEUKOPENIA

PNEUMONIA

OTITIS MEDIA

INTESTINAL INFLUENZA

SINUSITIS

0 1 2 3 4 5 6 7 8 9 10 11 12 13

INCUBATION (ALL TYPES)

ATTACK (EPIDEMIC)

SEQUELAE (ENDEMIC & PANDEMIC)

— EPIDEMIOLOGY —

VIRUS UNKNOWN + RESPIR-ATORY BACTERIA

Endemic – Every winter

VIRUSES A, B AND Y

Epidemic – Every second winter

VIRUS UNKNOWN + RESPIR-ATORY BACTERIA

Pandemic – Occurrence regular

16

SYMPTOMS

SYSTEMIC

The incubation period is 1 to 3 days.

The onset is sudden with chills, fever, discomfort, generalized pain and sometimes convulsions.

The temperature falls in a few days.

There is usually anorexia, vomiting or diarrhea.

The blood shows an early polymorphonuclear count followed by a leukopenia with monocytosis.

RESPIRATORY

Generalized manifestations converge to coryza, pharyngitis, tonsillitis, stomatitis, bronchitis.

They are out of all proportion to the local symptoms.

The severity of the attack diminishes in a few days unless bronchopneumonia develops.

Pulmonary edema and cyanosis predominate with hemorrhagic exudate in alveoli due to hemolytic streptococci or Pfeiffer's bacilli.

There may be otitis media, cervical lymphadenitis tracheobronchitis and laryngeal croup.

Development of pneumonia and other serious complications is due to secondary infection with pneumococci, hemolytic streptococci or Pfeiffer's bacillus.

Interstitial bronchopneumonia is due to the streptococcus.

Lobar pneumonia is due to the pneumococcus.

Pneumonia with abscess formation is due to the staphylococcus.

Resistance to secondary invasion is lowered because the virus conditions respiratory epithelium to further infection.

GASTRO-INTESTINAL

Sudden anorexia, abdominal pain, prostration and diarrhea do not necessarily warrant a diagnosis of intestinal grippe unless the condition is epidemic.

The stools contain mucus and occasionally blood.

There may be intestinal toxemia with little digestive disturbance.

The attack usually lasts several days but may be protracted.

NERVOUS

High fever, delirium, stupor and convulsions often suggest meningitis.

GASTROINTESTINAL MANIFESTATIONS OF INFLUENZA

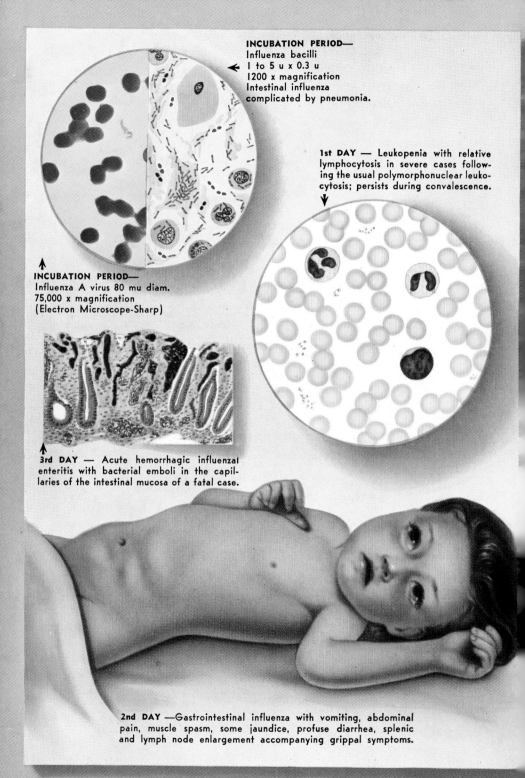

INCUBATION PERIOD—
Influenza bacilli
1 to 5 u x 0.3 u
1200 x magnification
Intestinal influenza
complicated by pneumonia.

INCUBATION PERIOD—
Influenza A virus 80 mu diam.
75,000 x magnification
(Electron Microscope-Sharp)

1st DAY — Leukopenia with relative lymphocytosis in severe cases following the usual polymorphonuclear leukocytosis; persists during convalescence.

3rd DAY — Acute hemorrhagic influenzal enteritis with bacterial emboli in the capillaries of the intestinal mucosa of a fatal case.

2nd DAY —Gastrointestinal influenza with vomiting, abdominal pain, muscle spasm, some jaundice, profuse diarrhea, splenic and lymph node enlargement accompanying grippal symptoms.

INFLUENZA — *continued*

Other cases exhibit fever without localizing symptoms.

The dyspnea is of central origin.

Lesions of the cerebrospinal system develop as complications.

COMPLICATIONS

Pneumonia, obstructive emphysema, atelectasis develop during an attack or as a sequel.

Pleurisy may lead to empyema.

Otitis media may result in mastoiditis.

Cervical lymphadenitis is invariably present.

Urinary disorders such as cystitis, pyelitis, and nephritis are rare.

Cutaneous disorders such as herpes and urticaria are common.

Nervous disorders such as paralysis, chorea, encephalitis and cyanosis may develop.

Complications develop in only 5% of the cases in ordinary epidemics.

PATHOLOGY

Tracheal and bronchial mucosa is purple, swollen, soft, velvety.

Lungs are collapsed, purple, leathery in affected areas and pale and emphysematous in unaffected areas.

Bronchioles are filled with yellow thick fluid.

Blood vessels are congested with frothy red fluid.

Pleural surfaces are covered with fibrinous exudate.

Lymph nodes throughout the body are enlarged and soft.

Spleen is moderately enlarged and the pulp is soft.

Liver is slightly enlarged and soft.

Adrenal cortex reveals petechiae and ecchymoses.

DIAGNOSIS

Easy in the presence of an epidemic but difficult in sporadic cases.

There is sudden onset, severe prostration, infected conjunctivae, flushed face, dusky cyanosis, fleeting pains, moderate leukopenia.

Inoculation of nasal washings into ferrets reproduces the disease.

Neutralizing antibodies and complement fixation tests may be positive.

Hemophilus influenzae may be isolated in throat cultures as a secondary invader.

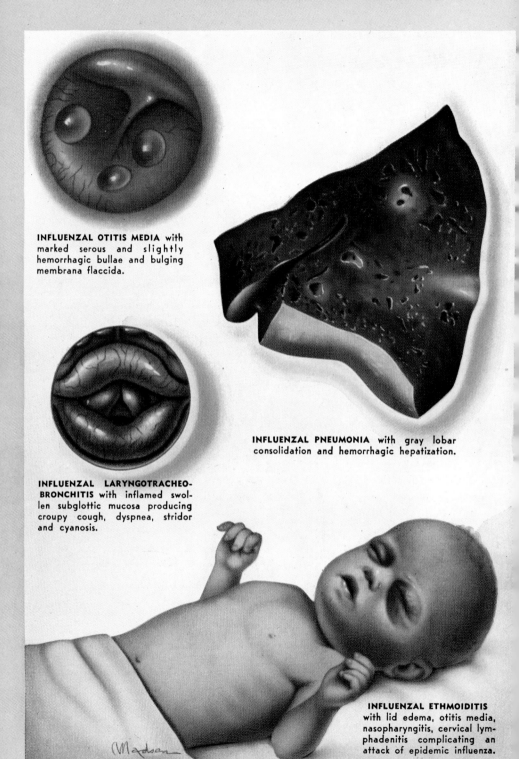

INFLUENZAL OTITIS MEDIA with marked serous and slightly hemorrhagic bullae and bulging membrana flaccida.

INFLUENZAL LARYNGOTRACHEO-BRONCHITIS with inflamed swollen subglottic mucosa producing croupy cough, dyspnea, stridor and cyanosis.

INFLUENZAL PNEUMONIA with gray lobar consolidation and hemorrhagic hepatization.

INFLUENZAL ETHMOIDITIS with lid edema, otitis media, nasopharyngitis, cervical lymphadenitis complicating an attack of epidemic influenza.

DIFFERENTIAL DIAGNOSIS

Common cold is characterized by less marked prostration.

Typhoid Fever is differentiated by laboratory tests in intestinal influenza.

Whooping Cough during the catarrhal stage may be diagnosed by marked leukocytosis.

Malaria may be detected by plasmodia in the blood.

Epidemic Myalgia is accompanied by localized pain in the lower chest or upper abdomen.

Miliary tuberculosis may be distinguished by roentgenogram, eye grounds and sputum examination.

Meningitis may be confirmed by lumbar puncture.

TREATMENT

Prophylactic antiviral rabbit serum by intranasal spray confers passive immunity. Influenza virus vaccine stimulates active immunity shortly before or even after onset of epidemic.

Influenza immunity may be expected within eight days following administration of nonviable vaccine.

Specific remedy is not available.

Convalescent serum from a person with high antibody titer is effective.

Rest in bed diminishes activity of the disease.

Isolation is necessary to protect the patient from other sources of infection.

Profuse perspiration may be decreased by tepid sponges.

Muscular aches may be overcome by light massage.

Nasopharyngeal irritation may be eased by hot gargles with Dobell's solution.

Nasal obstruction may be cleared by ephedrin drops or tampons. *Rhinalgan.*

Earache may be allayed by Auralgan without resorting to myringotomy.

Headache may be alleviated by ice cap and salicylates.

Cough may be eased by steam inhalation with tincture of benzoin.

Sleeplessness may be overcome by Dover's powder.

Early recognition and treatment of complications shortens the course.

General measures are instituted according to individual indications.

Sulfonamide or penicillin are indicated only after complications develop.

Adrenal cortex may abbreviate and alleviate postinfection asthenia during convalescence.

CEREBRAL COMPLICATIONS OF INFLUENZA

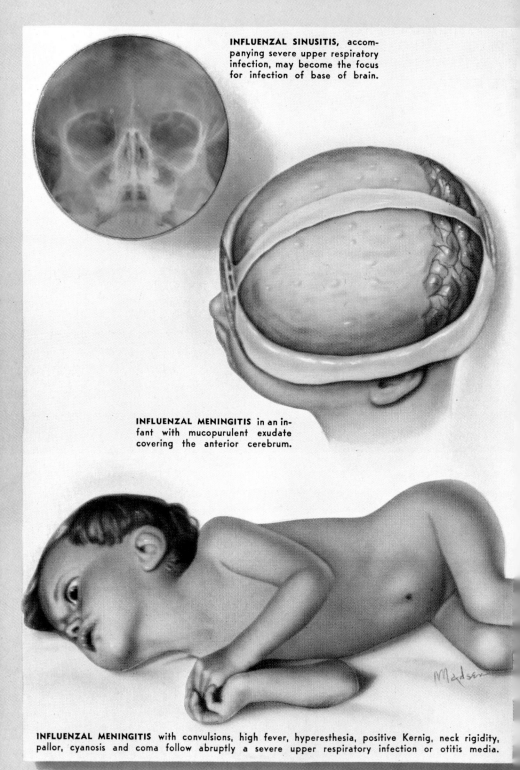

INFLUENZAL SINUSITIS, accompanying severe upper respiratory infection, may become the focus for infection of base of brain.

INFLUENZAL MENINGITIS in an infant with mucopurulent exudate covering the anterior cerebrum.

INFLUENZAL MENINGITIS with convulsions, high fever, hyperesthesia, positive Kernig, neck rigidity, pallor, cyanosis and coma follow abruptly a severe upper respiratory infection or otitis media.

REFERENCES:

FRANCIS, T., JR.: Transmission of Influenza by Filtrable Virus, *Science, 80:*457, Nov. 16, 1934.

SMITH, W., ANDREWES, C. H., and LAIDLAW, P. P.: Virus Obtained from Influenza Patients, *Lancet, 2:*66, July 8, 1933.

STOKES, J., JR., and others: Results of Immunization by Means of Active Virus of Human Influenza, *J. Clin. Investigation, 16:*237, March, 1937.

STOKES, J., JR., McGUINNESS, A. C., LANGNER, P. H., JR., and SHAW, D. R.: Vaccination Against Epidemic Influenza with Active Virus of Human Influenza: Two-Year Study, *Am. J. M. Sc., 194:*757, December, 1937.

STUART HARRIS, C. H., and others: A Study of Epidemic Influenza: With Special Reference to the 1936-7 Epidemic, Med. Research Council Special Rep. Ser. No. 228, p. 141. London, 1938, His Majesty's Stat. Office.

TAYLOR, R. M., and DREGUSS, M.: Experiment in Immunization Against Influenza with a Formaldehyde-Inactivated Virus, *Am. J. Hyg. Sect. B, 31:*31, January, 1940.

IV

M E A S L E S

(RUBEOLA)

NATURE

Measles is more widely prevalent than any other eruptive fever.

It is caused by a filtrable virus in the nasal and oral catarrhal secretions.

There is fever, cough, coryza, conjunctivitis, maculopapular eruption and Koplik spots.

The incubation period is 7 to 15 days after exposure to an infected individual.

It is followed by catarrhal symptoms for 4 days and a rash which lasts 6 days.

One attack confers a lifelong immunity since reinfection is rare.

ETIOLOGY

The causative filtrable virus is easily destroyed and not readily transmitted.

It does not persist in secretions for more than 2 weeks.

It is conveyed by direct contact, by the secretions, droplet infections, especially during the incubation period.

There are no long-time carriers during epidemics.

The disease is endemic in large cities in odd years and epidemic in even years.

It recurs in epidemic form after a few years during the winter and spring.

An infant born of a mother who has contracted measles before delivery develops the disease.

If a mother is exposed shortly before labor, both infant and mother develop the disease simultaneously.

Infants usually have an immunity during the first 5 months of life.

Thereafter susceptibility is greatest between 3 and 5 years of age.

SYMPTOMS

INCUBATION

This period lasts about 10 days when the catarrhal symptoms first appear.

There may, however, be catarrhal manifestations, febrile reactions and anorexia.

A leukopenia with reduction in lymphocytes develops in the course of incubation.

There may be irritability, fatigue, drowsiness, headache or convulsions.

INVASION

Onset is gradual with symptoms of a common cold.

There may be urticaria, erythema, buccal eruptions and conjunctivitis.

Then follow lacrimation, photophobia, coryza, sneezing and dry cough.

CLINICAL COURSE OF MEASLES

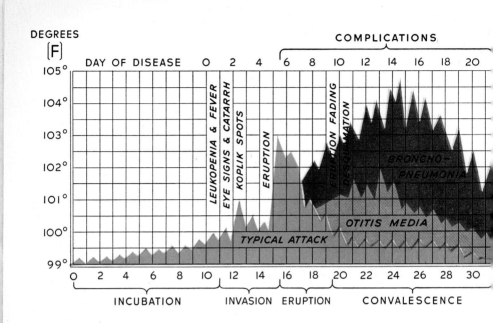

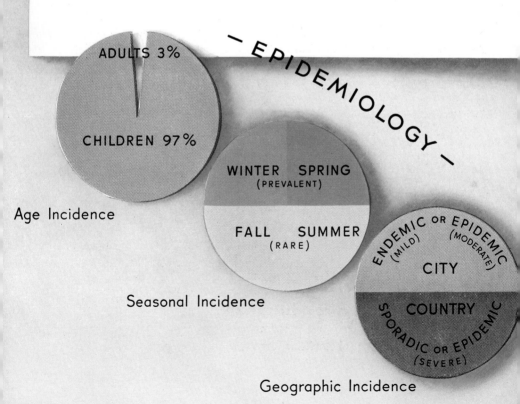

Age Incidence

Seasonal Incidence

Geographic Incidence

By the second or third day small red macules appear on the palate.
Koplik spots appear on the mucous membrane lining of the lips and cheeks.
The duration of the invasion is 3 to 4 days.

ERUPTION

The rash appears by the third or fifth day.
First it appears on the scalp, temples, behind the ears or on the neck.
Then, over the whole body except the legs, forearms, hands and feet.
Later, even the palms and soles become covered within 36 hours.
Individual spots reach a maximum development within 24 hours and then fade.
All traces disappear by the fifth day after the first appearance.
There remains a brownish pigmentation for several days.

DESICCATION

The eruptive and desiccative stages cannot be sharply defined.
The latter begins with the disappearance of the eruption on the fifth day followed by scaling until the tenth day.
It occurs first on the face and then elsewhere, in the order in which the eruption developed.

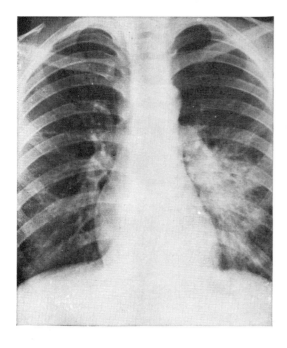

Bronchopneumonia is indicated by persistent fever, accelerated respiratory rate, sudden prostration, accompanied by dullness, bronchial breathing and fine rales. Infants and young children may show pneumonic infiltration during the eruptive or post-eruptive period without definite physical signs.

DEVELOPMENT OF MEASLES

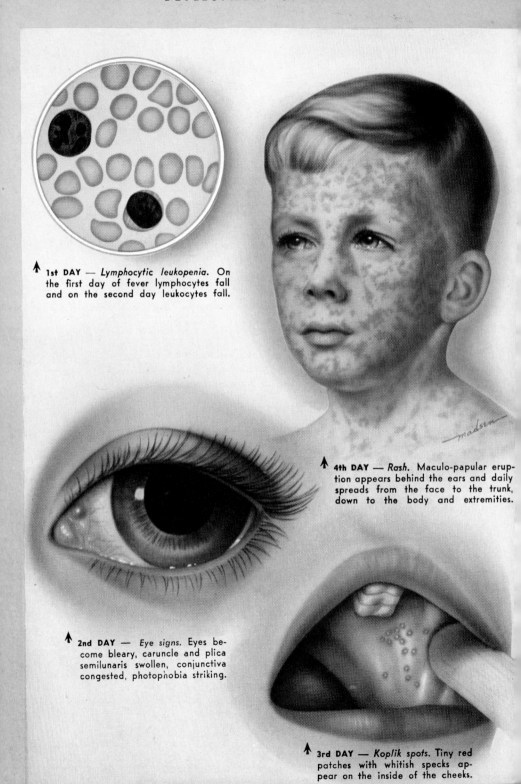

1st DAY — *Lymphocytic leukopenia.* On the first day of fever lymphocytes fall and on the second day leukocytes fall.

4th DAY — *Rash.* Maculo-papular eruption appears behind the ears and daily spreads from the face to the trunk, down to the body and extremities.

2nd DAY — *Eye signs.* Eyes become bleary, caruncle and plica semilunaris swollen, conjunctiva congested, photophobia striking.

3rd DAY — *Koplik spots.* Tiny red patches with whitish specks appear on the inside of the cheeks.

COMPLICATIONS

Otitis media may be catarrhal or suppurative, evidenced by recurrent fever, ear pain, redness and bulging drum.
It develops in the eruptive stage and may lead to mastoiditis and meningitis.
Infants may develop purulent otitis without other evidence than discharge from the ear during the late eruptive stage.
Bronchopneumonia develops in the eruptive stage as the most fatal complication.
Lobar pneumonia is much less common but empyema may follow either.
Failure of the temperature to fall after full appearance of the rash may indicate respiratory complications especially laryngotracheobronchitis and bronchopneumonia.
Laryngitis may become ulcerative or even develop into diphtheria.
Cervical lymphadenitis occurs in conjunction with throat complications.
Encephalitis may develop within a week after the onset of the rash.
It is characterized by a mental condition varying from apathy to stupor or delirium.

DIAGNOSIS

During the period of invasion Koplik spots are pathognomonic.
The rash is visible under ultraviolet light before it can otherwise be detected.
Leukopenia is the rule but in severe cases leukocytosis may appear during the incubation period.
Inclusion bodies may be demonstrated in smears of the nasal mucosa.
Intracutaneous injection of convalescent serum will abort development of a rash in that area.

PROPHYLAXIS

Intramuscular injection of convalescent serum within 7 days after exposure.
It provides immunity for 3 weeks or prevents measles.
Modified measles develops if serum is given 7 to 14 days after exposure.
Whole blood 1 or 2 ounces intramuscularly or intravenously is less efficacious.
Immune globulin 2 to 4 cc. injected intramuscularly modifies the course of the disease in 75% of cases if given before appearance of rash.

TREATMENT

Nonspecific and symptomatic under complete isolation for 2 weeks.
Immune transfusions or convalescent serum are helpful in severe cases.
Dark glasses relieve excessive photophobia.
Auralgan relieves earache by arresting inflammation.
Steam inhalation with menthol alleviates laryngitis.
Calamine lotion over the skin alleviates itching.
Early recognition of complications calls for appropriate treatment.
Sulfonamide or penicillin for prophylaxis against bacterial complications.

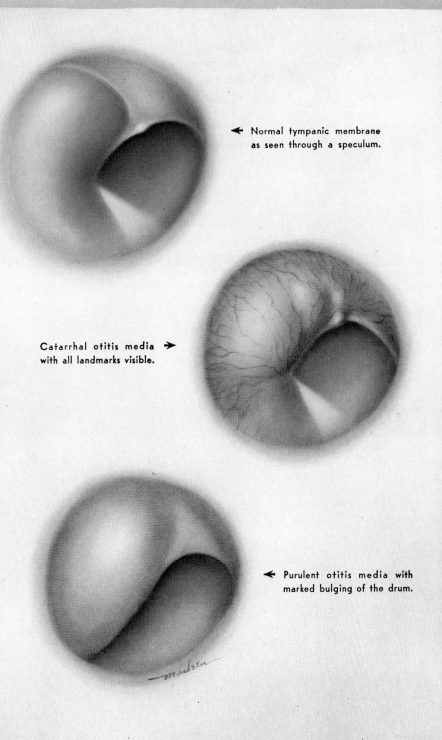

← Normal tympanic membrane
as seen through a speculum.

Catarrhal otitis media →
with all landmarks visible.

← Purulent otitis media with
marked bulging of the drum.

REFERENCES:

BRINCKER, J. A. H.: A Historical, Epidemiological and Aetiological Study of Measles, *Proc. Roy. Soc. Med., 31:*807, 1938.

DENTON, J.: The Pathology of Fatal Measles, *Am. J. M. Sc., 169:*531, 1925.

ENDERS, J. F.: The Etiology of Measles, in Virus and Rickettsial Diseases, Cambridge, Harvard Univ. Press, 1940.

HAMILTON, P. M., and HANNA, R. J.: Encephalitis Complicating Measles, *Am. J. Dis. Child., 61:*483, 1941.

JANEWAY, C. A.: Use of Concentrated Human Serum Gamma Globulin in the Prevention and Attenuation of Measles, *Bull. New York Acad. Med., 21:*202, 1945.

KOPLIK, H.: A New Diagnostic Sign of Measles, *Med. Rec., 53:*505, 1898.

McKHANN, C. F.: The Prevention and Modification of Measles, *J.A.M.A., 109:* 2034, 1937.

PETERMAN, M. G., and FOX, M. J.: Postmeasles Encephalitis, *Am. J. Dis. Child., 57:*1253, 1939.

RAKE, GEOFFREY: Experimental Investigation of Measles, *J. Pediat., 23:*376, 1943.

SHAFFER, M. F., RAKE, G., and HODES, H. L.: Isolation of Virus from a Patient with Fatal Encephalitis Complicating Measles, *Am. J. Dis. Child., 64:*815, 1942.

STILLERMAN, M., MARKS, H. H., and THALHIMER, WM.: Prophylaxis of Measles with Convalescent Serum, *Am. J. Dis. Child., 67:*1, 1944.

WARTHIN, A. S.: Occurrence of Numerous Large Giant Cells in the Tonsils and Pharyngeal Mucosa in the Prodromal Stage of Measles, *Arch. Path., 11:*864, 1931.

WEISBECKER: Heilserum gegen Masern, *Ztschr. f. klin. Med., 30:*312, 1896.

WESTWATER, J. S.: Tuberculin Allergy in Acute Infectious Diseases: Study of Intracutaneous Test, *Quart. J. Med., 4:*203, 1935.

V

M U M P S
(EPIDEMIC PAROTITIS)

NATURE

Swelling of the salivary glands, particularly the parotids is accompanied by mild constitutional symptoms.

Other glandular structures, particularly the testes, may be affected in adults.

Infants are rarely affected although everyone is susceptible.

It is most common between 5 and 15 years of age, especially during the winter and spring.

ETIOLOGY

The causative agent is a filtrable virus demonstrated in the blood stream and saliva of affected children.

Incubation period varies from 12 to 21 days.

Transmitted by contact with infected case, secretions or soiled articles.

Communicability from onset to disappearance of glandular enlargement.

Immunity following an attack may be lifelong.

IMMUNITY

Natural immunity is nonexistent except during the first eight months.

The newborn may develop the disease if the mother is not immune.

Passive immunity may be induced early by convalescent serum.

One attack tends to confer permanent immunity.

Recurrence in a previously affected individual is not rare.

SYMPTOMS

Invasion for a day or two simulates a mild infection.

There is pain, stiffness at the angle of the jaws in front of ears.

There is marked swelling in the region of the parotid gland.

Swelling is first on one side and in 2 or 3 days on the other.

The skin is not red, the pain moderate, the fever high.

Pain is increased by swallowing cold or sour substances.

The openings of Stensen's ducts are swollen.

Saliva becomes scanty, the mouth dry and the tongue furred.

CLINICAL COURSE OF MUMPS

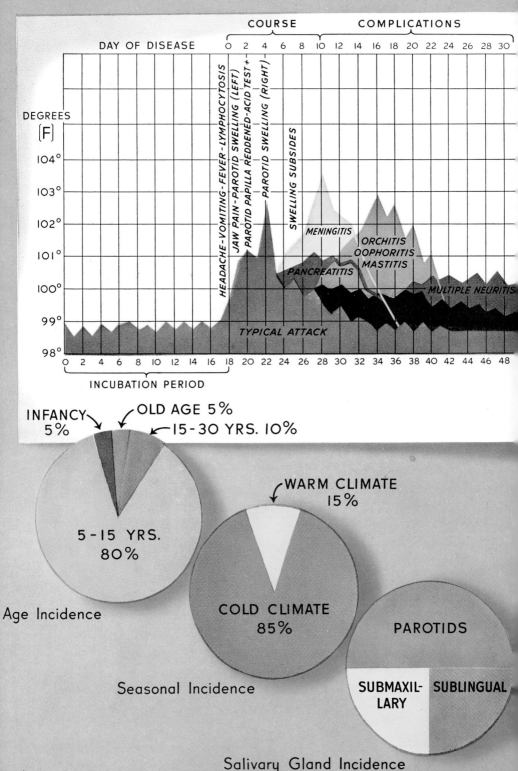

COURSE   COMPLICATIONS

DAY OF DISEASE   0 2 4 6 8 10 12 14 16 18 20 22 24 26 28 30

DEGREES
(F)

104°

103°

102°

101°

100°

99°

98°

HEADACHE - VOMITING - FEVER - LYMPHOCYTOSIS

JAW PAIN - PAROTID SWELLING (LEFT)

PAROTID PAPILLA REDDENED - ACID TEST +

PAROTID SWELLING (RIGHT)

SWELLING SUBSIDES

MENINGITIS

ORCHITIS
OOPHORITIS
MASTITIS

PANCREATITIS

MULTIPLE NEURITIS

TYPICAL ATTACK

0 2 4 6 8 10 12 14 16 18 20 22 24 26 28 30 32 34 36 38 40 42 44 46 48

INCUBATION PERIOD

INFANCY
5%

OLD AGE 5%

15 - 30 YRS. 10%

5 - 15 YRS.
80%

Age Incidence

WARM CLIMATE
15%

COLD CLIMATE
85%

Seasonal Incidence

PAROTIDS

SUBMAXIL-
LARY   SUBLINGUAL

Salivary Gland Incidence

34

MUMPS — *continued*

Enlargement of the neighboring lymphatic glands is usually present.

Suppuration never occurs, hence the differentiation from suppurative parotitis.

Swelling of the glands disappears in 10 days.

The blood shows a lymphocytosis.

COMPLICATIONS

ORCHITIS

It is rare under 10 years of age, probably not more than 1%.

It develops in the second week especially on the right side.

There is testicular pain, tenderness and severe constitutional reaction.

When the swelling subsides, atrophy or destruction of the testicle tends to follow but impotence and sterility are not common.

In girls, the breast and vulva may be involved and ovaries destroyed.

Rest, support, cool applications and locally 50% methyl salicylate in lanolin.

PANCREATITIS

It may develop at the end of the first week.

There is prostration, digestive disturbances, abdominal pain for a week.

The urine remains sugar-free.

MENINGO-ENCEPHALITIS

It is a rare complication except during epidemics.

Meningeal irritation and high fever develop toward end of first week.

There is sudden fever, headache, neck rigidity and positive Kernig.

Mental changes and delirium may be evident from onset.

Spinal fluid is under increased pressure but clear.

There is predominance of lymphocytes but normal sugar content.

Most cases recover spontaneously and death is a rarity.

Meningeal symptoms may be relieved by daily lumbar puncture.

TREATMENT

During the febrile course the child should be kept in bed in isolation.

Pain may be alleviated by hot fomentations or belladonna ointment.

A fluid diet of all cooked and strained foods will obviate painful chewing.

Mouth hygiene is essential to prevent secondary infection of the parotid.

Orchitis may be prevented by injection of 10 cc. of convalescent serum.

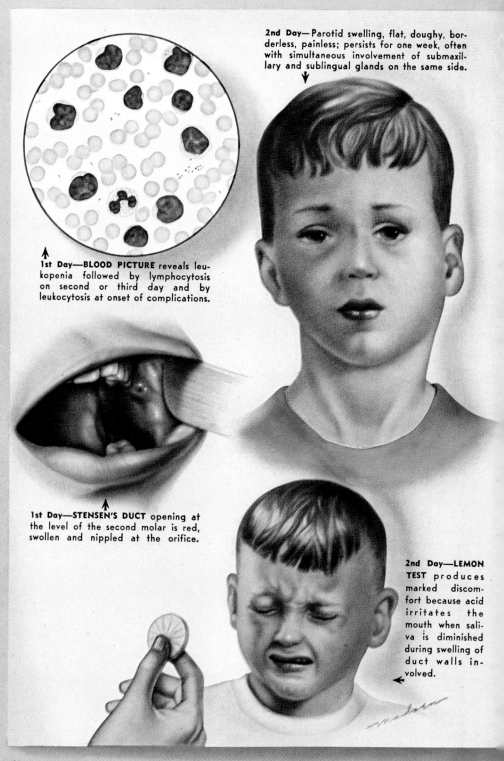

2nd Day—Parotid swelling, flat, doughy, borderless, painless; persists for one week, often with simultaneous involvement of submaxillary and sublingual glands on the same side.

1st Day—BLOOD PICTURE reveals leukopenia followed by lymphocytosis on second or third day and by leukocytosis at onset of complications.

1st Day—STENSEN'S DUCT opening at the level of the second molar is red, swollen and nippled at the orifice.

2nd Day—LEMON TEST produces marked discomfort because acid irritates the mouth when saliva is diminished during swelling of duct walls involved.

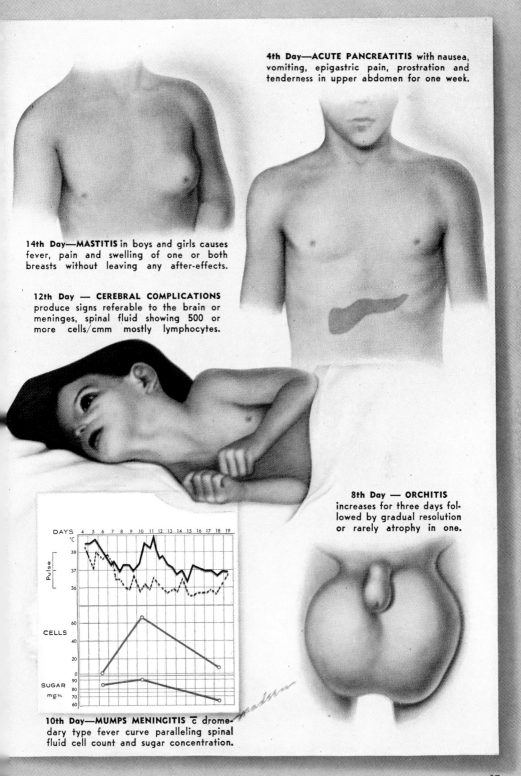

4th Day—ACUTE PANCREATITIS with nausea, vomiting, epigastric pain, prostration and tenderness in upper abdomen for one week.

14th Day—MASTITIS in boys and girls causes fever, pain and swelling of one or both breasts without leaving any after-effects.

12th Day — CEREBRAL COMPLICATIONS produce signs referable to the brain or meninges, spinal fluid showing 500 or more cells/cmm mostly lymphocytes.

8th Day — ORCHITIS increases for three days followed by gradual resolution or rarely atrophy in one.

10th Day—MUMPS MENINGITIS c̄ drome-dary type fever curve paralleling spinal fluid cell count and sugar concentration.

REFERENCES:

BRAHDY, M. B., and SCHEFFER, I. H.: Pancreatitis Following Mumps, *Am. J. M. Sc., 181:*255, 1931.

BIRNBERG, T. L.: Mumps Meningo-Encephalitis, *Minnesota Med., 22:*145, 1939.

ENDERS, J. F.: Techniques of Laboratory Diagnosis, Tests for Susceptibility and Experiments on Specific Prophylaxis, *J. Pediat., 29:*129, 1946.

FINKELSTEIN, HERMAN: Meningo-Encephalitis in Mumps, *J.A.M.A., 111:*17, 1938.

GELLIS, S. S., McGUINNESS, A. C., and PETERS, M.: A Study on the Prevention of Mumps Orchitis by Gamma Globulin, *Am. J. Dis. Child., 210:*661, 1945.

GORDON, J. E.: Epidemiology of Mumps, *Am. J. M. Sci., 200:*412, 1940.

HABEL, KARL: Cultivation of Mumps Virus in the Developing Chick Embryo, *Pub. Health Rep., 60:*201, 1945.

HOLDEN, E. M., EAGLES, A. Y., STEVENS, J. E., JR.: Mumps Involvement of the Central Nervous System, *J.A.M.A., 131:*382, 1946.

MONTGOMERY, J. C.: Mumps Meningo-Encephalitis, *Am. J. Dis. Child., 48:*1279, 1934.

RAMBAR, A. C.: Mumps, Use of Convalescent Serum in the Treatment and Prophylaxis of Orchitis, *Am. J. Dis. Child., 71:*1, 1946.

WESSELHOEFT, C.: Mumps: Its Glandular and Neurologic Manifestations, in Virus and Rickettsial Diseases, Cambridge, Harvard Univ. Press, 1940, p. 309.

VI

PERTUSSIS
(WHOOPING COUGH)

NATURE

Whooping cough is an acute contagious disease of the respiratory tract caused by the bacillus pertussis.

It is characterized by spasmodic attacks of hard coughing which end with a typical respiratory whoop and expulsion of a stringy tenacious mucus from the trachea.

ETIOLOGY

The causative bacillus Bordet-Gengou is a small hemophilic gram-negative organism.

It is found in children with pertussis and occasionally in persons associated with them.

Transmission is by direct exposure and not by carriers.

The disease is endemic in cities.

Epidemics occur in winter and spring often in association with measles.

Incubation period is from 7 to 14 days.

Newborns are highly susceptible to the disease and to its complications.

One attack protects the child throughout life.

SYMPTOMS

CATARRHAL

The attack begins with tracheobronchitis, malaise and irritability.

The cough becomes hard, dry and disturbing especially at night.

After a fortnight of febrile catarrhal state, the paroxysmal period develops.

PAROXYSMAL

Explosive expiratory coughs develop suddenly followed by a long drawn inspiration and a crowing sound.

The face becomes cyanosed, the eyes blood-shot and the child runs for help. A typical whoop consists of a severe long expiratory cough with a long inspiratory crow which continues until a plug of mucus is dislodged.

CONVALESCENT

After a month of paroxysms the whoop ceases and the cough resembles an ordinary bronchitis.

This stage continues for 3 weeks but may be prolonged indefinitely in winter.

Even after it ceases the whoop may return with an attack of bronchitis but it must not be considered a relapse of pertussis.

It is merely a habit pattern of paroxysmal coughing which passes after months of diminishing practice.

CLINICAL COURSE OF PERTUSSIS

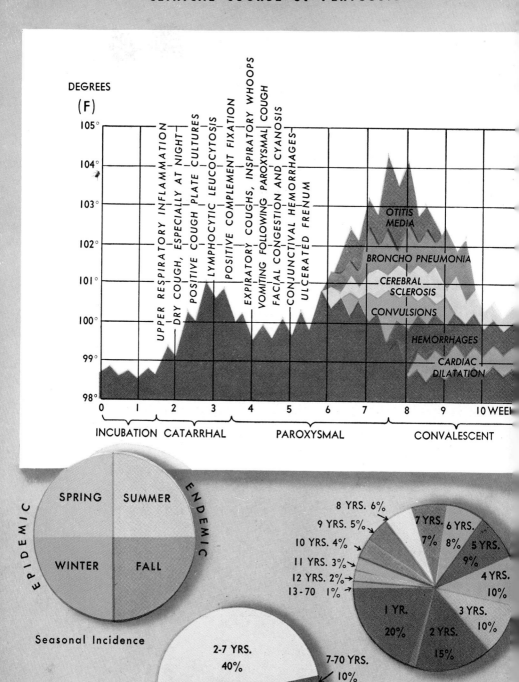

DEGREES (F)

105°
104°
103°
102°
101°
100°
99°
98°

UPPER RESPIRATORY INFLAMMATION
DRY COUGH, ESPECIALLY AT NIGHT
POSITIVE COUGH PLATE CULTURES
LYMPHOCYTIC LEUCOCYTOSIS
POSITIVE COMPLEMENT FIXATION
EXPIRATORY COUGHS, INSPIRATORY WHOOPS
VOMITING FOLLOWING PAROXYSMAL COUGH
FACIAL CONGESTION AND CYANOSIS
CONJUNCTIVAL HEMORRHAGES
ULCERATED FRENUM

OTITIS MEDIA
BRONCHO PNEUMONIA
CEREBRAL SCLEROSIS
CONVULSIONS
HEMORRHAGES
CARDIAC DILATATION

0 1 2 3 4 5 6 7 8 9 10 WEEI

INCUBATION CATARRHAL PAROXYSMAL CONVALESCENT

EPIDEMIC   ENDEMIC

SPRING SUMMER
WINTER FALL

Seasonal Incidence

8 YRS. 6%
9 YRS. 5%
10 YRS. 4%
11 YRS. 3%
12 YRS. 2%
13 - 70 1%

7 YRS. 7%   6 YRS. 8%   5 YRS. 9%

4 YRS. 10%

1 YR. 20%   2 YRS. 15%   3 YRS. 10%

Mortality Incidence

2-7 YRS. 40%   7-70 YRS. 10%

Age Incidence

40

© 1949 - AURALGAN - OTOSMOSA

PERTUSSIS — *continued*

COMPLICATIONS

RESPIRATORY

Bronchopneumonia is more frequent in young children.
It occurs at the height of the paroxysmal stage.
Atelectasis is common due to blocking of a bronchus with mucus.
Emphysema is always present and may remain as a sequel.
Otitis media follows infection of the nasopharynx.

DIGESTIVE

Vomiting invariably follows the paroxysms.
There may be anorexia, stomatitis, indigestion and rectal prolapse.
Gastric tetany may follow alkalosis due to loss of gastric acid secretions.

NERVOUS

Asphyxia from paroxysms may lead to convulsions that may also be due to tetany or to cerebral hemorrhage.
Other types are due to serous meningitis or encephalitis.
A rare complication is cortical degeneration or the so-called progressive cerebral sclerosis.

DIAGNOSIS

Cough plates contain a spray from the child's mouth during coughing.
Incubated for 3 days they reveal pearl-like colonies of pertussis organisms.
Blood counts during early paroxysmal stage show marked leukocytosis with predominance of lymphocytes.
Blood sedimentation rate is retarded while in other infections it is accelerated.

PROPHYLAXIS

Passive immunization may be given by intramuscular injections of 10-30 cc of hyperimmune serum or convalescent serum or 5-10 cc of immune rabbit serum.
Active immunity may be developed by injecting infants with 7 cc. of 15 billion pertussis bacilli per cc. hypodermatically.
3 injections are given at 3 week intervals consisting of 1 cc., 2 cc. and 4 cc. respectively.

TREATMENT

Sulfadiazine, codein, chloral and phenobarbital control the paroxysms.
25% of ether in oil may be injected rectally in 1 oz. retentions to diminish spasm and induce sleep.
After vomiting, feedings should be repeated.
Small meals between spasms are preferable to 3 meals a day.
Thick feeding for infants and solid food for children will be retained.

TYPICAL ATTACK OF PERTUSSIS

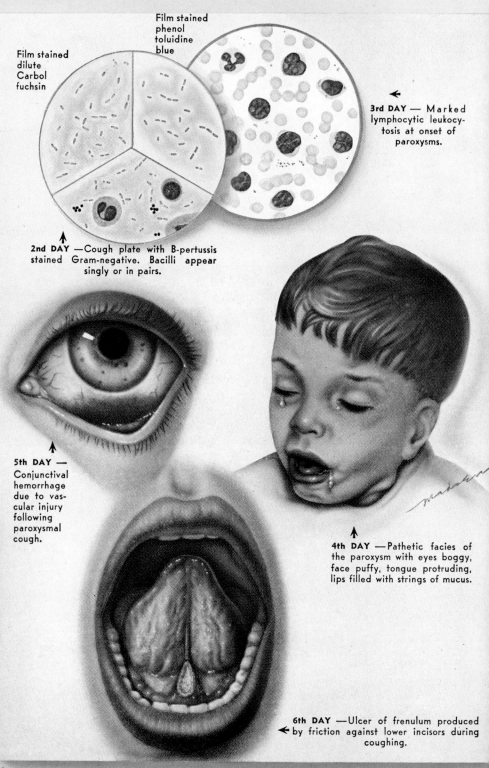

Film stained phenol toluidine blue

Film stained dilute Carbol fuchsin

3rd DAY — Marked lymphocytic leukocytosis at onset of paroxysms.

2nd DAY — Cough plate with B-pertussis stained Gram-negative. Bacilli appear singly or in pairs.

5th DAY — Conjunctival hemorrhage due to vascular injury following paroxysmal cough.

4th DAY — Pathetic facies of the paroxysm with eyes boggy, face puffy, tongue protruding, lips filled with strings of mucus.

6th DAY — Ulcer of frenulum produced by friction against lower incisors during coughing.

COMPLICATIONS OF PERTUSSIS

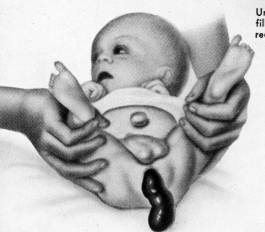

Umbilical hernia is mushroom shaped filled with omentum while anal and rectal prolapse reveals sigmoid flexure and colon.

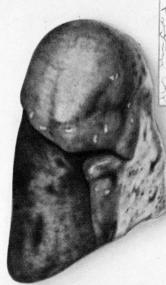

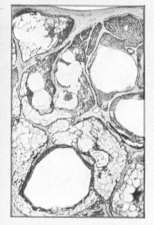

Bronchiectasis during severe pertussis or after recovery revealed by an area at the base with persistent rales changed by expectoration.

Pulmonary Emphysema occurs in severe cases and clears with convalescence. It is observed in every case of pertussis at autopsy.

Pneumonitis due to B-pertussis or other organisms develops at the close of the spasmodic stage.

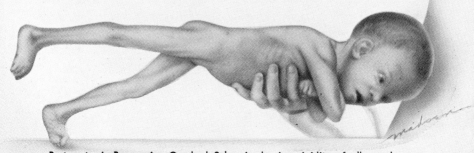

Post-pertussis Progressive Cerebral Sclerosis showing rigidity of all muscles.

REFERENCES:

BORDET, J., and GENGOU, O.: Le Microbe de la coqueluche, *Ann. Inst. Pasteur,* 20:731, 1906.

BRADFORD, W. L., DAY, E., and BERRY, G. P.: Improvement of the Nasopharyngeal Swab Method of Diagnosis in Pertussis by the Use of Penicillin, *Am. J. Pub. Health, 36:*468, 1946.

DOLGOPOL, V. B.: Changes in the Brain in Pertussis with Convulsions, *Arch. Neurol. and Psychiat., 46:*477, 1941.

FELTON, H. M.: The Status of Passive Immunization and Treatment in Pertussis Vaccine, *J.A.M.A., 126:*294, 1944.

FLOSDORF, E. W., FELTON, H. M., BONDI, A., and McGUINNESS, A. C.: Intradermal Test for Susceptibility to and Immunization Against Whooping Cough Using Agglutinogen from Phase I. H. Pertussis, *Am. J. M. Sc., 206:*422, 1943.

HABEL, KARL, and LUCCHESI, P. F.: Convulsions Complicating Pertussis, *Am. J. Dis. Child., 56:*275, 1938.

KENDRICK, P., THOMPSON, M., and ELDERING, G.: Immunity Response of Mothers and Babies to Infections of Pertussis Vaccine During Pregnancy, *Am. J. Dis. Child., 70:*24, 1945.

KOH, J. L., SCHWARTZ, I., GREENBAUM, J., and DALY, M. M. I.: Roentgenograms of the Chest Taken During Pertussis, *Am. J. Dis. Child., 67:*463, 1944.

LAPIN, J. H.: Immunization Against Whooping Cough, *J. Pediat., 29:*90, 1946.

MACDONALD, H., and MACDONALD, E. J.: Experimental Pertussis, *J. Infect. Dis., 53:*328, 1933.

McGUINNESS, A. C., ARMSTRONG, J. G., and FELTON, H. M.: Hyperimmune Whooping Cough Serum, *J. Pediat., 24:*249, 1944.

MILLER, J. J., HUMBER, J. B., and DOWRIE, J. O.: Immunizations with Combined Diphtheria and Tetanus Toxoids (Aluminum Hydroxide Absorbed) Containing Hemophilus Pertussis Vaccine, *J. Pediat., 24:*281, 1944.

RICH, A. R.: On the Etiology and Pathogenesis of Whooping Cough, *Bull. Johns Hopkins Hosp., 51:*346, 1932.

SAKO, W., TREUTING, W., WITT, D., and NICHAMIN, S.: Early Immunization Against Pertussis with Alum Precipitated Vaccine, *J.A.M.A., 127:*379, 1945.

SAUER, L. W., and MARKLEY, E. D.: Whooping Cough: Pertussis Agglutinogen Skin Test After Immunization with Hemophilus Pertussis Vaccine, *J.A.M.A., 131:*967, 1946.

SEARS, W. G.: The Nervous Complications of Whooping Cough, *Brit. J. Child. Dis., 26:*178, 1929.

SEITZ, R. P.: Extreme Leukocytosis in Pertussis, *Am. J. Dis. Child., 30:*670, 1925.

SILVERTHRONE, NELLES: Whooping Cough, *J. Pediat., 25:*584, 1944.

VII

POLIOMYELITIS
(INFANTILE PARALYSIS)

NATURE

Acute virus infection with sudden onset, fever and malaise gives rise to myelitis with or without flaccid paralysis of various muscle groups.

ETIOLOGY

Virus enters gastrointestinal tract in food and water contaminated by flies and insects.

Infection passes on to the central nervous system via sympathetic and parasympathetic pathways.

EPIDEMIOLOGY

Direct contact with human carriers transmits the disease.

Virus persists in nasopharynx and feces for months.

Incubation period is 7 to 10 days.

Babies are not susceptible because of maternal antibodies.

Second attacks are rare.

It occurs from July to October.

Incidence is highest in rural regions, lowest in the tropics.

Fleas, insects, pests and animals are carriers.

Fecal contamination of food and water transmit the virus.

Tonsillectomized children are more susceptible during epidemics.

SYMPTOMS

SPINAL TYPE

First day

Onset is abrupt like an acute infection.

There is vomiting, constipation and fever.

Drowsiness, irritability, headache and prostration.

Second day

Hyperasthenia, rigidity of neck or extremities, pain on motion.

Head is supported with difficulty, spine is rigid.

Third day

Fever subsides, symptoms abate.

Paralysis progressive, posture dorsal.

Opisthotonos common; deep reflexes, increased, then lost.

Pain on motion or pressure.

Urinary retention; persistent constipation.

BULBOSPINAL TYPE

Onset is abrupt like acute infection.

Symptoms are severe as in spinal type.

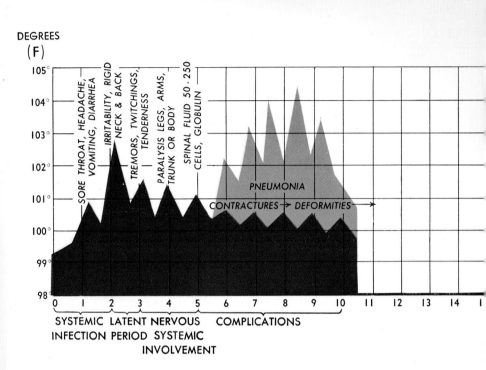

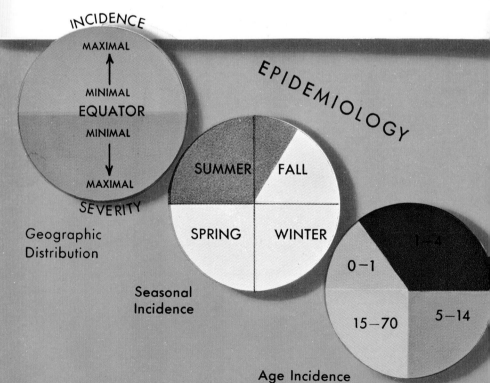

POLIOMYELITIS — *continued*

Bulbar paralysis is unilateral or bilateral.
Facial paralysis is transient.
Ocular paralysis causes internal strabismus.
Speech disturbance is transient.
Impaired swallowing necessitates tube feeding.
Other paralyses occur in neck, diaphragm, intercostals or upper extremities.
Exitus is due to respiratory paralysis, circulatory failure or pneumonia.

ABORTIVE TYPE
Prodromal symptoms simulate acute infections.
Virus is present in nasal washings and stools.
Prevalent during epidemics.
Paralysis never develops.
Spinal fluid, if examined, is typical.

PROPHYLAXIS

Avoid fatigue, exercise, chilling, swimming.
Avoid contact with groups, carriers, flies.
Inject 20 cc. convalescent serum, 40 cc. gamma globulin or 60 cc. pooled blood.

COURSE

Spontaneous improvement after acute stage.
Muscular power improves within one year.
Residual paralysis is permanent.
Atrophy of paralyzed muscles.
Growth of affected limb is arrested.
Deformities prevalent depend on site of involvement.

LABORATORY

BLOOD
Moderate leukocytosis, increased polymorphonuclears.

SPINAL FLUID
Slightly opalescent, pressure increased.
Cells 50 to 250 or more.
Polymorphonuclears predominate at first, globulin is increased later.
Sugar is normal.

TREATMENT

Complete rest of affected parts and isolation for 3 weeks from onset.
Discharges from nose and mouth should be disinfected.
Prophylactic serum 20 cc. intramuscularly is slightly beneficial.
Warm packs are applied over affected musculature by Kenny method.
Lumbar punctures relieve increased intracranial pressure.
Muscle spasm may be alleviated by neostigmin and curare intramuscularly.
Pain may be relieved by Demerol 25 mgm. q. 3 hrs.

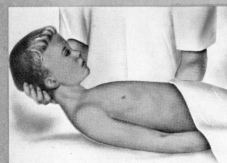

STIFF NECK — patient resists flexion of the neck.

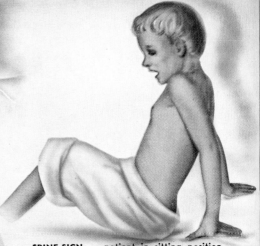

SPINE SIGN — patient in sitting position holds his back stiff supported with his arms behind.

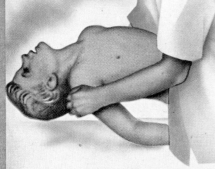

HEAD DROP — patient's head falls backward when his shoulders are lifted.

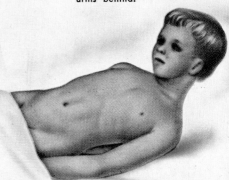

UMBILICAL SIGN — patient with paralysis of lower abdominal wall muscles moves the umbilicus upward when raising his head.

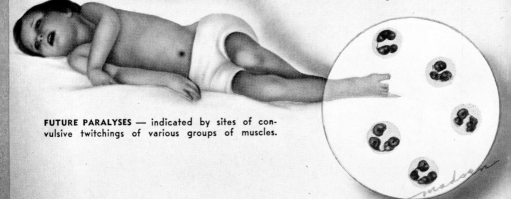

FUTURE PARALYSES — indicated by sites of convulsive twitchings of various groups of muscles.

SPINAL FLUID — shows increased pressure, increased protein and increased cells mostly polymorphonuclears.

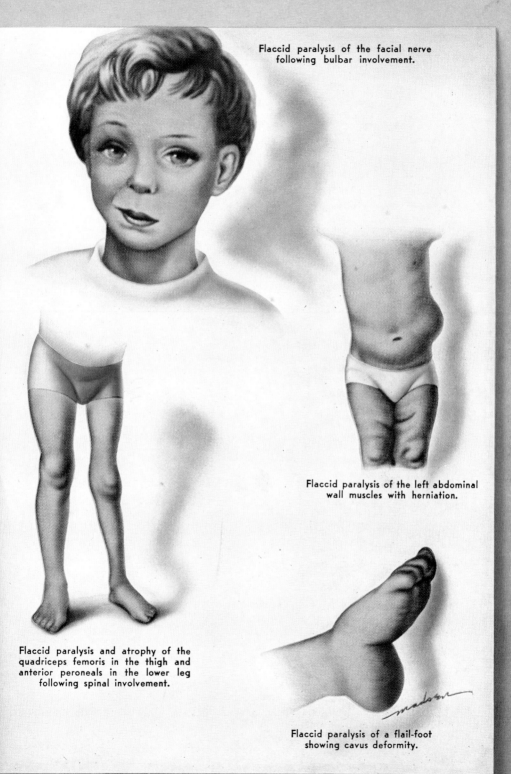

Flaccid paralysis of the facial nerve following bulbar involvement.

Flaccid paralysis of the left abdominal wall muscles with herniation.

Flaccid paralysis and atrophy of the quadriceps femoris in the thigh and anterior peroneals in the lower leg following spinal involvement.

Flaccid paralysis of a flail-foot showing cavus deformity.

Bulbar paralysis requires postural drainage with frequent shifting, suction with aspirator, atropin as needed.
Tube feeding and parenteral fluid may be necessary.
Oxygen tent and Drinker respirator may be life-saving.

REFERENCES:

AMERICAN ORTHOPEDIC ASSOCIATION: Infantile Paralysis or Acute Poliomyelitis, *J.A.M.A., 131:*1411, 1946.

ANDERSON, J. A.: Poliomyelitis and Recent Tonsillectomy, *J. Pediat., 27:*68, 1945.

AYCOCK, W. L., and LUTHER, E. H.: Preparalytic Poliomyelitis, *J.A.M.A., 91:*387, 1928.

BAHLKE, A. M., and PERKINS, J. E.: Treatment of Preparalytic Poliomyelitis with Gamma Globulin, *J.A.M.A., 129:*1146, 1945.

BENNETT, R. L.: The Role of Physical Medicine in Poliomyelitis, *J. Pediat., 28:* 316, March, 1946.

BILLIG, H. E., JR.: Muscle Reinnervation, *J. Internat. Coll. Surgeons, 7:*457, 1944.

BRIDGE, E. W.: The Diagnosis of Abortive Poliomyelitis, *J. Pediat., 29:*597, 1946.

DANIELS, LUCILLE, WILLIAMS, MARIAN, and WORTHINGHAM, CATHERINE: Muscle Testing: Techniques of Manual Examination, Philadelphia, W. B. Saunders Co., 1946.

DRINKER, P., and McKHANN, C. F.: The Use of a New Apparatus for the Prolonged Administration of Artificial Respiration, *J.A.M.A., 92:*1658, 1929.

DUBLIN, W. B., BADE, B. A., and BROWN, B. A.: Pathologic Findings in Nerve and Muscle in Poliomyelitis, *Am. J. Clin. Path., 14:*266, 1944.

GUREWITSCH, A. D., and O'NEILL, M. A.: Hot Baths in the Treatment of Early Poliomyelitis, *J. Pediat., 28:*554, 1946.

HOWE, H. A., and BODIAN, D.: Neural Mechanisms in Poliomyelitis, New York, The Commonwealth Fund, 1942.

KABAT, H., and KNAPP, M. E.: The Use of Prostigmine in the Treatment of Poliomyelitis, *J.A.M.A., 122:*989-995, 1943.
The Mechanism of Muscle Spasm in Poliomyelitis, *J. Pediat., 24:*123-137, 1944.

NATIONAL FOUNDATION FOR INFANTILE PARALYSIS: Pub. No. 45, A Guide for Nurses in the Nursing Care of Patients with Infantile Paralysis, New York, 1945.

PAUL, J. R., SALINGER, R., and TRASK, J. D.: Abortive Poliomyelitis, *J.A.M.A., 98:* 2262, 1932.

POHL, J. F., and KENNY, ELIZABETH: The Kenny Concept of Infantile Paralysis, Minneapolis, Bruce Pub. Co., 1943.

QUIGLEY, T. B.: Second Attacks of Poliomyelitis, *J.A.M.A., 102:*752, 1934.

SCHLESINGER, E. B.: Recent Advances in the Use of Curare in Clinical Practice, *Bull. New York Acad. Med., 22:*520, 1946.

SCHWARTZ, R. P., BOUMAN, H. D., and SMITH, W. K.: The Significance of Muscle Spasm, *J.A.M.A., 126:*695, 1944.

STEINDLER, ARTHUR: The Newer Pathological and Physiological Concepts of Anterior Poliomyelitis and Their Clinical Interpretation, *J. Bone and Joint Surg., 29:*59, 1947.

WARD, R., MELNICK, J. L., and HORSTMANN, D. M.: Poliomyelitis Virus in Fly-Contaminated Food Collected at an Epidemic, *Science, 101:*491, 1945.

WRIGHT, JESSIE: Problems in Early Treatment of Poliomyelitis, *New York State J. Med., 44:*67, 1944.

VIII

RUBELLA
(GERMAN MEASLES)

NATURE

German measles is a contagious eruptive fever.

It is rarely seen except epidemically.

It is characterized by a short period of invasion with mild constitutional symptoms.

There is upper respiratory catarrh, swelling of posterior cervical lymph nodes and eruption of diffusely rose-colored macules.

One attack confers life-long immunity.

ETIOLOGY

The causative filtrable virus is present in the secretions of the nose and throat.

It is transmitted by direct contact but rarely by fomites or a third person.

The greatest incidence is in winter and early spring.

Infants under 6 months show a striking immunity.

The incubation period is 14 to 21 days.

Infectivity is maximal for a day or two before the eruption appears.

SYMPTOMS

The onset is sudden with small, pale red macular papulous rash.

It varies in size from a pin-head to a pea, discrete or confluent.

The rash appears first on the face or neck, around the mouth or behind the ears.

It extends within a day to the whole body.

A few spots may be seen in the mouth.

After 1 to 3 days desquamation may develop.

There may be fever, cervical lymphadenopathy, sore throat and mild constitutional disturbances.

Complications are rare although otitis, arthritis, nephritis, encephalitis or meningo-encephalitis may develop in a severe epidemic.

Cataract, patent ductus arteriosus and other congenital anomalies may appear in an infant born of a mother who had rubella during the first three months of pregnancy.

Convalescence is rapid.

TREATMENT

Symptomatic care will suffice.

The patient should be kept in bed until all symptoms subside.

Quarantine ceases after seven days.

Pooled human serum controls epidemics.

CLINICAL COURSE OF RUBELLA

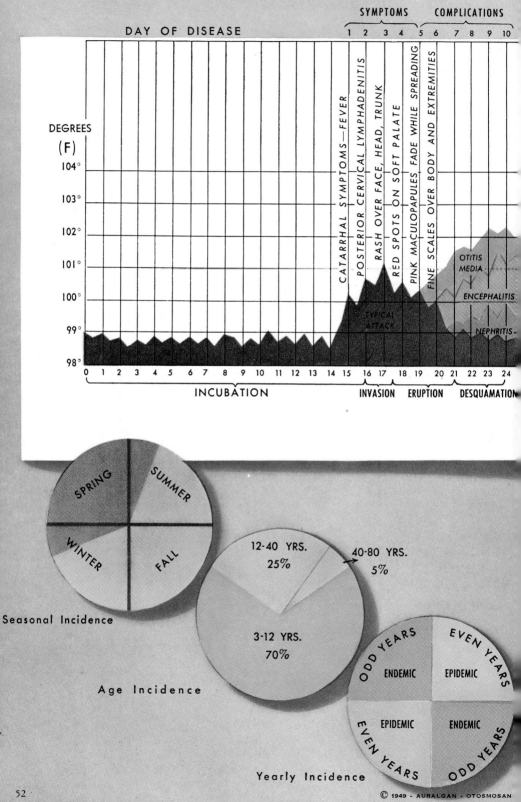

SYMPTOMS   COMPLICATIONS

DAY OF DISEASE   1 2 3 4 5 6 7 8 9 10

CATARRHAL SYMPTOMS—FEVER
POSTERIOR CERVICAL LYMPHADENITIS
RASH OVER FACE, HEAD, TRUNK
RED SPOTS ON SOFT PALATE
PINK MACULOPAPULES FADE WHILE SPREADING
FINE SCALES OVER BODY AND EXTREMITIES

DEGREES (F)
104°
103°
102°
101°
100°
99°
98°

OTITIS MEDIA
ENCEPHALITIS
NEPHRITIS

TYPICAL ATTACK

0 1 2 3 4 5 6 7 8 9 10 11 12 13 14 15 16 17 18 19 20 21 22 23 24

INCUBATION   INVASION ERUPTION DESQUAMATION

Seasonal Incidence

SPRING   SUMMER
WINTER   FALL

Age Incidence

12-40 YRS. 25%   40-80 YRS. 5%
3-12 YRS. 70%

Yearly Incidence

ODD YEARS ENDEMIC   EVEN YEARS EPIDEMIC
EVEN YEARS EPIDEMIC   ODD YEARS ENDEMIC

CLINICAL FEATURES OF RUBELLA

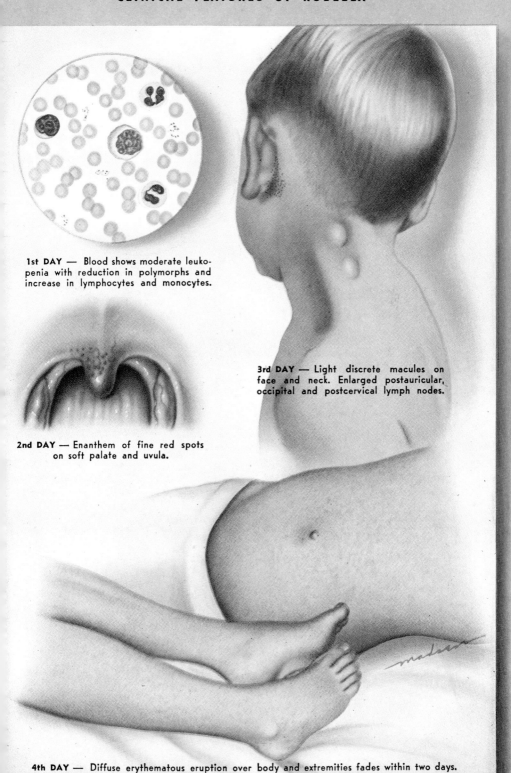

1st DAY — Blood shows moderate leukopenia with reduction in polymorphs and increase in lymphocytes and monocytes.

2nd DAY — Enanthem of fine red spots on soft palate and uvula.

3rd DAY — Light discrete macules on face and neck. Enlarged postauricular, occipital and postcervical lymph nodes.

4th DAY — Diffuse erythematous eruption over body and extremities fades within two days.

REFERENCES:

ALBAUGH, C. H., Congenital Anomalies Following Maternal Rubella in Early Weeks of Pregnancy, *J.A.M.A., 129:*719, 1945.

CARRIEU, LAMY, and BOUCHET: La roubeole n'est pas toujours une maladie benigne, *Presse. méd., 36:*274, 1938.

CARROLL, J. V.: The Blood Count in Rubella with Special Reference to Plasma Cells and Turk Cells, *Lancet, i:*182, 1934.

CLEMENS, H. H.: Exanthem Subitum, *J. Pediat., 26:*66, 1945.

CONTE, W. R., MCCAMMON, C. S., and CHRISTIE, AMOS: Congenital Defects Following Maternal Rubella, *Am. J. Dis. Child., 70:*301, 1945.

DAVISON, CHARLES, and FRIEDFELD, LOUIS: Acute Encephalomyelitis Following German Measles, *Am. J. Dis. Child., 55:*496, 1938.

ELEY, R. C.: Neurologic Conditions in Infants and Children, *J. Pediat., 7:*261, 1935.

GOTTLIEB, JULIUS: Placental Extract in the Control of German Measles, *Maine M. J., 27:*10, 1936.

GRAHAM, J. R.: Rubella, *New York State J. Med., 32:*1368, 1932.

GREGG, N. M.: Congenital Cataract Following German Measles in the Mother, *Tr. Ophth. Soc. Australia,* (1941), *3:*35, 1942.

MARGOLIS, F. J., WILSON, J. L., and TOP, F. H.: Postrubella Encephalomyelitis, *J. Pediat., 23:*158, 1943.

OWEN and GREENWAY: Meningo-encephalitis Following Rubella, *M. J. Australia, 2:*536, 1940.

REESE, A. B.: Congenital Cataract and Other Anomalies Following Rubella, *Am. J. Ophth., 27:*483, 1944.

SOMERSET, W. L.: The Diagnosis of German Measles, *Weekly Bull. Dept. of Health, City of New York, 13:*202, 1924.

TEITAL, D.: Exanthema Subitum, *Arch. de méd. d. enf., 32:*327, 1929.

TEMPLETON, H. J., and SUTHERLAND, R. T.: The Exanthem of Acute Mononucleosis, *J.A.M.A., 113:*1215, 1939.

ZAHORSKY, J.: Roseola Infantum, *J.A.M.A., 61:*1446, 1913.

IX

SCARLET FEVER
(SCARLATINA)

NATURE
Scarlatina is caused by many types of group A hemolytic streptococci. It is characterized by a sudden sore throat, an erythematous eruption and a tendency to otitis media, lymphadenitis and nephritis.

ETIOLOGY
The causative organism is one of several group A beta-hemolytic streptococci. It is transmitted by direct contact with one suffering from the disease or by contact with carriers, discharges, fomites, contaminated milk or food.

Incubation period is 2 to 5 days, invasion 12 to 24 hours and desquamation 3 to 6 weeks.

The pharynx is the usual portal of entry.

Infants under one year of age rarely contract the disease, even from an infected mother. Children between two and seven years of age are most susceptible.

White children are far more susceptible than colored.

Certain families have particular immunity.

The disease is rare in the tropics, endemic in temperate zones and epidemic at 5 year intervals, especially in girls during the winter and fall.

TYPES
SIMPLE . . . Tonsillitis is followed by manifestation of toxin absorption. Enlargement of the cervical lymph glands and transient albuminuria are common.

TOXIC . . . Toxin production and absorption may be overwhelming. Onset is marked by rigors, high fever, vomiting, diarrhea and delirium. The rash is profuse and dusky.

SEPTIC . . . Local or general sepsis, due to the specific or allied organism, is superimposed upon the toxemia, especially in young children. Bronchopneumonia often terminates the disease.

SYMPTOMS
INVASION . . . Onset is abrupt with vomiting, high fever and sore throat. Erythematous blush covers the pharynx, tonsils and fauces with red points over the hard palate.

Convulsions may develop in very young children.

ERUPTION . . . A red rash like a uniform blush appears from 12 to 36 hours or later after the onset.

It blanches in mild cases and becomes hemorrhagic in severe cases.

Petechiae appear by tourniquet test.

Face and scalp are devoid of rash.

Itching, burning or even swelling appear at the height of the eruption.

CLINICAL COURSE OF SCARLET FEVER

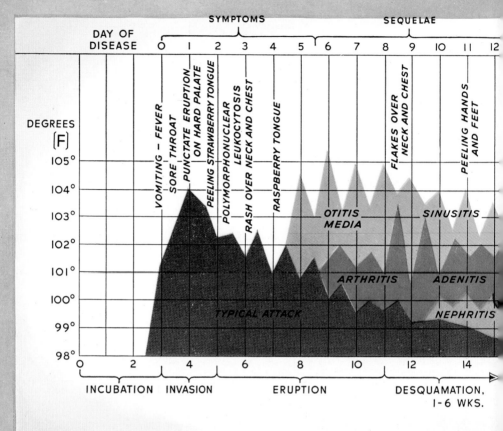

SYMPTOMS | SEQUELAE

DAY OF DISEASE: 0 1 2 3 4 5 6 7 8 9 10 11 12

DEGREES (F): 105° 104° 103° 102° 101° 100° 99° 98°

VOMITING – FEVER
SORE THROAT
PUNCTATE ERUPTION ON HARD PALATE
PEELING STRAWBERRY TONGUE
POLYMORPHONUCLEAR LEUKOCYTOSIS
RASH OVER NECK AND CHEST
RASPBERRY TONGUE
FLAKES OVER NECK AND CHEST
PEELING HANDS AND FEET

OTITIS MEDIA
SINUSITIS
ARTHRITIS
ADENITIS
NEPHRITIS
TYPICAL ATTACK

0 2 4 6 8 10 12 14

INCUBATION | INVASION | ERUPTION | DESQUAMATION, 1-6 WKS.

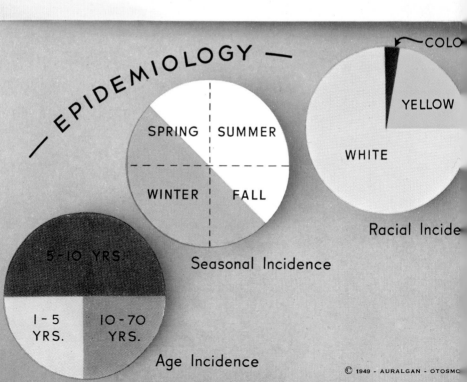

— EPIDEMIOLOGY —

SPRING | SUMMER
WINTER | FALL

Seasonal Incidence

COLO...
YELLOW
WHITE

Racial Incide...

5-10 YRS.
1-5 YRS.
10-70 YRS.

Age Incidence

56

ENANTHEM . . . Initial congestion of the pharynx, tonsils and fauces gives way to a fine blush or membranous inflammation when the skin eruption appears. Submucous hemorrhage develops over the palate.

The tongue is heavily coated on the first day, clear at the tip on the second day and anteriorly on the third, giving the characteristic strawberry appearance.

DESQUAMATION . . . When the rash fades about the eighth day, the neck and chest shed fine flakes.

Desquamation of the trunk is complete within 3 weeks unless baths are given, especially over thick epidermis of the hands and feet.

Skin shedding continues for 2 months.

COMPLICATIONS

CERVICAL ADENITIS . . . Slight swelling occurs in most cases during the first few days.

Marked swelling occurs in severe throat involvements.

It proceeds to abscess formation, cellulitis or convalescence.

OTITIS MEDIA . . . A suppurative process may develop on the second day or later, especially in infants.

There is marked destruction of the tympanic cavity leading to deafness or more immediately to mastoiditis.

NEPHRITIS . . . Febrile albuminuria early in the disease is of short duration.

Acute nephritis develops at the end of the third week in mild or severe cases. Onset is gradual or abrupt.

ARTHRITIS . . . Joint pains may occur with the development of the rash as a toxic manifestation or as a result of serum sickness from specific therapy.

Polyarthritis is of rheumatic origin.

Suppurative arthritis of pyemic origin follows scarlet fever and usually involves the large joints.

SEPTICEMIA . . . Presence of the hemolytic streptococcus in the blood is responsible for protracted septic fever, general toxicity, stormy convalescence or exitus.

DIAGNOSIS

CLINICAL . . . Abrupt onset, vomiting, high fever, erythematous throat, punctate palate, raspberry tongue, history of exposure, throat culture positive for beta-hemolytic streptococci and finally desquamation.

DICK TEST . . . Inject intradermally 0.2 cc. 1:1,000 filtrate of broth culture from scarlatinal streptococcus.

A change from a positive reaction in the first days of disease to a negative during convalescence indicates that the condition was scarlatinal.

A persistently positive test casts doubt upon the diagnosis.

SCHULTZ-CARLTON REACTION . . . Intracutaneous injection of 0.2 cc. of potent therapeutic serum brings about a rapid blanching of a recent scarlet fever rash.

CLINICAL FEATURES OF SCARLET FEVER

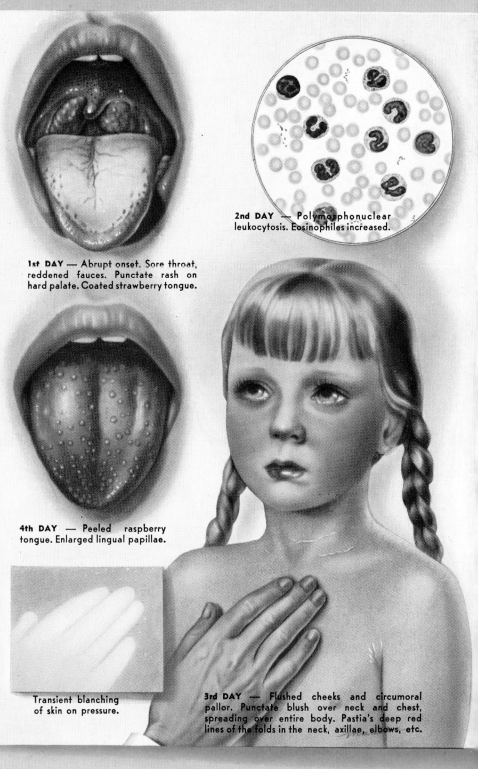

1st DAY — Abrupt onset. Sore throat, reddened fauces. Punctate rash on hard palate. Coated strawberry tongue.

2nd DAY — Polymorphonuclear leukocytosis. Eosinophiles increased.

4th DAY — Peeled raspberry tongue. Enlarged lingual papillae.

Transient blanching of skin on pressure.

3rd DAY — Flushed cheeks and circumoral pallor. Punctate blush over neck and chest, spreading over entire body. Pastia's deep red lines of the folds in the neck, axillae, elbows, etc.

SCARLET FEVER — continued

A positive result is pathognomonic, but a negative result is indeterminate in 24 hours.

PROPHYLAXIS

QUARANTINE . . . Two negative throat cultures for streptococcus scarlatinae are the best criteria for release from a 4 week quarantine.
About 3% become permanent carriers.

ACTIVE IMMUNIZATION . . . Infants one year of age and older children with a positive Dick test should be given 5 weekly injections of 500, 2,000, 8,000, 25,000, and 90,000 skin test doses respectively of scarlet fever toxin.
A Dick test should be done 2 months later to determine the efficacy of the immunization.
If positive, re-immunization is necessary.
Half the immunized children lose their immunity in 1 year.

PASSIVE IMMUNIZATION . . . Injection of convalescent serum 5 to 10 cc. intramuscularly after exposure is protective.
Serum obtained from Dick-negative donors is effective in doses of 30 cc.
Placental extract is indefinite.
Antitoxin in doses of 2,000 units is preventive but it produces reactions.

TREATMENT

ANTITOXIN . . . Severe cases require a single intramuscular injection of 6,000 units. If no improvement is evident the dose is repeated in 24 hours.
In toxic cases the serum is given intravenously.
A test for serum sensitivity must be made in advance.
If sensitive, desensitization must be carried out.

SERUM . . . Pooled convalescent serum gives no reaction and is more efficacious than antitoxin.
It may be given intramuscularly or intravenously in doses of 50 cc.
Normal serum of Dick-negative donors and blood transfusions are also beneficial.

SULFONAMIDE . . . The daily oral dose varies from 15 grs. for infants to 50 grs. for older children given in divided doses at 4 hour intervals.
Addition of equal amounts of sodium bicarbonate prevents development of acidosis from the drug especially in complications such as otitis media, cervical adenitis, mastoiditis, septicemia, etc. Penicillin also reduces complications.

DRUGS . . . Sore throat is relieved by irrigation with mild antiseptic solution.
Discharging nose may be cleared by sulfathiazole-ephedrine drops. *Rhinalgan.*
Congested ear drums may be alleviated by Auralgan.
Restlessness may be overcome by antipyretic drugs.
Itchy skin may be soothed by 1% thymol or 2% antihistaminic ointment.
Toxic states with cyanosis require caffein or digitalis hypodermically.

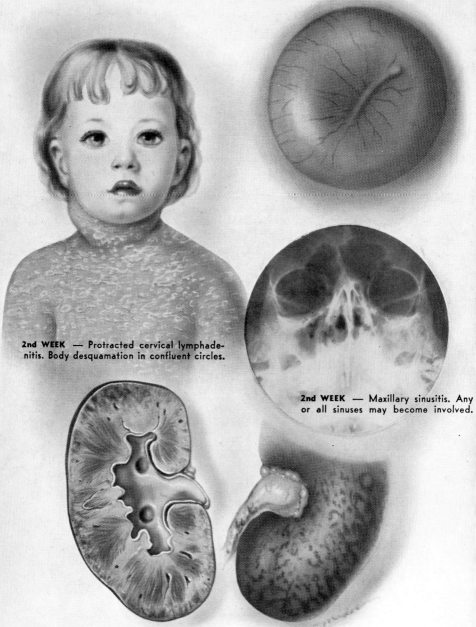

1st WEEK — Acute suppurative otitis. Reddened bulging tympanic membrane.

2nd WEEK — Protracted cervical lymphadenitis. Body desquamation in confluent circles.

2nd WEEK — Maxillary sinusitis. Any or all sinuses may become involved.

3rd WEEK — Acute hemorrhagic glomerulonephritis. Urine scanty, reddish-brown with considerable albumin, red blood cells, blood pigments and possibly pus cells.

SCARLET FEVER — continued

REFERENCES:

Ashley, Paul: The Treatment of Scarlet Fever, *J.A.M.A., 130:*771, 1946.

Best, William H.: A Study of Secondary Cases of Scarlet Fever, *New York State J. Med., 33:*881, 1933.

Dick, G. F., and Dick, G. H.: A Scarlet Fever Antitoxin, *J.A.M.A., 82:*1246, April 19, 1924.

Dochez, A. R., and Sherman, L.: The Significance of Streptococcus Hemolyticus in Scarlet Fever and the Preparation of a Specific Anti-scarlatinal Serum by Immunization of the Horse to Streptococcus Hemolyticus Scarlatinae, *J.A.M.A., 82:*542, February 16, 1924.

Hoyne, A. L., Levinson, S. C., and Thalhimer, William: Convalescent Scarlet Fever Serum, *J.A.M.A., 105:*783, 1935.

Joe, A.: Scarlatinal Arthritis, *Edinburgh M. J., 31:*341, 1924.

Kiskaddon, R. M.: An Epidemiological Study of Scarlet Fever, *Arch. Pediat., 58:* 624 and 706, 1941.

Lancefield, R. C.: A Serological Differentiation of Human and Other Groups of Hemolytic Streptococci, *J. Exper. Med., 57:*571, 1933.

Lovett, B. R.: Scarlet Fever Following Nose and Throat Operations, *J.A.M.A., 87:*96, 1926.

Peacock, S., Bigler, J. A., and Werner, Marie: Scarlet Fever, Hemolytic Streptococcic Cultures and Dick Tests in Children's Hospital, *Am. J. Dis. Child., 57:* 759, 1939.

Rolleston, J. D.: Return Cases of Scarlet Fever and Their Prevention, *Brit. J. Child. Dis., 29:*91, 1932.

Thalhimer, William: The Use of Convalescent Scarlet Fever and Measles Sera in Prophylaxis and Therapy, *Bull. New York Acad. Med., 14:*361, 1938.

Veldee, M. V.: Preparation of a Scarlet Fever Streptococcus Toxoid and Its Use in Active Immunization, *Pub. Health Rep., 48:*549, 1933.

Watson, R. F., Schwentker, F. F., Fetherston, J. E., and Rothbard, S.: Sulfadiazine Prophylaxis in an Epidemic of Scarlet Fever, *J.A.M.A., 122:*730, 1943.

Wesselhoeft, Conrad: Cardiovascular Disorders in Scarlet Fever, *New England J. Med., 224:*942, 1941.

X

SMALLPOX
(VARIOLA)

NATURE

Variola is characterized by a 3-day febrile period.
It is followed by a generalized eruption which passes through stages of papule, vesicle, pustule and crust.
There is renewed constitutional disturbance at the time of pustulation.
A tendency to secondary infection by the streptococcus is invariable.

ETIOLOGY

An infant may contract smallpox in utero.
It may be infected at the time of birth.
Maternal vaccination does not protect the infant.
Epidemics occur in the winter and spring.
The virus is transmitted by direct contact, fomites, insects or by a carrier.
One attack confers lasting immunity.

PATHOLOGY

Apart from the specific lesions there is nothing characteristic.
There is myocardial degeneration, cloudy swelling and focal necrosis.
There is also fatty degeneration of the liver and kidneys and necrotic change in other viscera responsible for their enlargement.

SYMPTOMS

INCUBATION
The period ranges between 10 and 13 days without symptoms.
When the disease is acquired by inoculation into the skin, the incubation is shorter.

INVASION
Onset is sudden with fever.
Then follows vomiting, diarrhea, generalized pain, headache or convulsions.
As the fever rises there is restlessness, sleeplessness and often delirium.

ERUPTION
The rash develops first on the face and forearms.
Then on the upper arms and trunk.
On the third day the rash spreads over the lower extremities.
Skinfolds, axillae and groins are spared.
The lesions are macular, then papular, then hard.
Vesiculation begins about the periphery spreading toward the center.
The fully developed vesicle content becomes purulent.
The pustule ruptures about the tenth day and forms crusts.

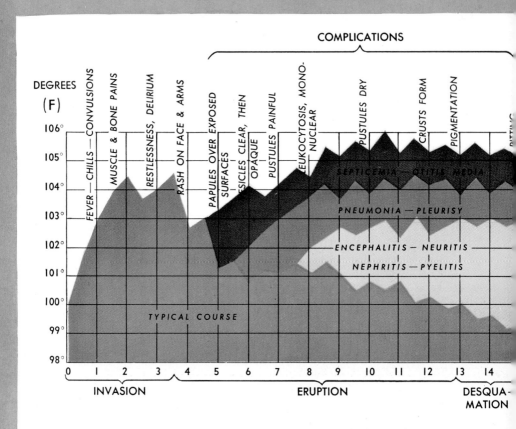

COMPLICATIONS

DEGREES (F)

FEVER — CHILLS — CONVULSIONS
MUSCLE & BONE PAINS
RESTLESSNESS, DELIRIUM
RASH ON FACE & ARMS
PAPULES OVER EXPOSED SURFACES
VESICLES CLEAR, THEN OPAQUE
PUSTULES PAINFUL
LEUKOCYTOSIS, MONO-NUCLEAR
PUSTULES DRY
CRUSTS FORM
PIGMENTATION
PITTING

106°
105°
104°
103°
102°
101°
100°
99°
98°

SEPTICEMIA — OTITIS MEDIA
PNEUMONIA — PLEURISY
ENCEPHALITIS — NEURITIS
NEPHRITIS — PYELITIS

TYPICAL COURSE

0 1 2 3 4 5 6 7 8 9 10 11 12 13 14

INVASION | ERUPTION | DESQUA-MATION

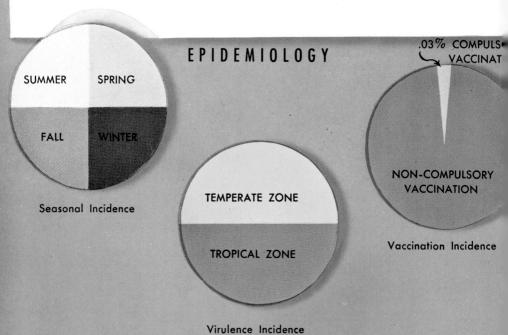

EPIDEMIOLOGY

SUMMER | SPRING
FALL | WINTER

Seasonal Incidence

TEMPERATE ZONE
TROPICAL ZONE

Virulence Incidence

.03% COMPULS- VACCINAT

NON-COMPULSORY VACCINATION

Vaccination Incidence

TYPES

CONFLUENT

The lesions fuse.
Constitutional symptoms are severe.
Delirium and prostration are the rule.

HEMORRHAGIC

Purpuric rash appears giving the body a purplish hue.
Hemorrhages from mucous membranes develop.
The true eruption tends to be obliterated.
The hemorrhagic tendency may be manifest in the vesicles or pustules.

VARIOLOID

This modified form of the disease occurs in children partially protected
by vaccination.
The disease clears on the fourth day after rapid progression of the eruptive
stages.

COMPLICATIONS

SKIN

There may be impetigo, boils, abscesses, erysipelas.

SENSES

Conjunctivitis occurs in severe cases.
Keratitis, followed by destruction of the globe may result in blindness.
Otitis media is not uncommon.

CARDIAC

Myocardial failure may occur at any stage but most commonly during pustulation.

RESPIRATORY

Laryngeal lesions may lead to edema of the glottis.
Bronchitis is usual and bronchopneumonia common.

DIAGNOSIS

EYE TEST

A needle dipped in a pustule is used for scarifying the cornea of a rabbit.
In smallpox, vesicular lesions appear on the cornea in 48 hours and proceed
to necrosis.
Histological examination reveals Guarnieri's inclusion bodies.

COMPLEMENT FIXATION TEST

This reaction is used with specific immune serum from inoculated animals.
Pock fluid gives positive results.

FLOCCULATION TEST

Saline extracts from the crust of a suspected case are used.
Various dilutions of a rabbit vaccinia flocculating serum are added.
Occurrence of flocculation after incubation is confirmatory.

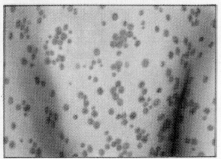

1st DAY — Round rose-colored macules resembling measles become embedded firm papules.

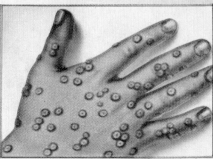

4th DAY — Multilocular vesicles with depressed grayish centers form over the papules.

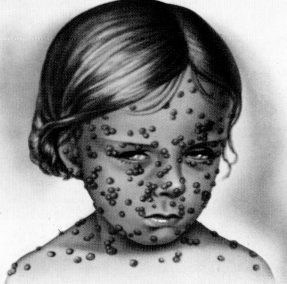

7TH DAY — Globular yellowish pustules form from the enlarging umbilicated vesicles.

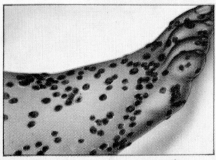

10th DAY —Brownish crusts form from dried pustules with dark centers leaving bluish areas.

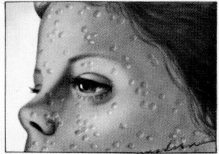

15th DAY —Permanent pitting follows confluent but not discrete smallpox.

SMALLPOX — *continued*

VACCINATION TEST

Vaccination is given after the onset of an eruption in an unvaccinated child.
It will fail to react if the eruption is smallpox.

PROPHYLAXIS

ACTIVE IMMUNITY

Primary vaccination gives immunity for 5 to 10 years.
All children except those with eczema should be vaccinated before the sixth month of life.
Press the side of a needlepoint rapidly into a drop of virus onto the upper arm or calf of the leg.
Virus may be wiped off and no dressings necessary until pustule forms.
In 6 to 10 days primary reaction develops in a nonimmune child.
In 4 to 7 days accelerated reaction develops in a partially immune child.
In 2 to 3 days a papule develops as an immune reaction.
It should be protected with sterile gauze for 3 weeks.
If no pustule forms in 2 weeks vaccination should be repeated until a take occurs.

PASSIVE IMMUNITY

Serum of vaccinated persons and of those convalescent from the disease can neutralize the virus.
Immune serum is valuable for rapid protection against smallpox.

TREATMENT

ISOLATION

Medical aseptic technique must be put into effect.
It serves against contact infection and against insect-borne and air-borne infections.
Disinfection of all discharges from the child must be rigidly observed.
All articles leaving the child's surroundings must be boiled for 30 minutes.
Isolation must be continued until all crusts have disappeared in 4 to 6 weeks.

SYSTEMIC

Fluids must be forced or given parenterally to prevent dehydration.
Convalescent serum is beneficial.
Sulfonamides and penicillin prevent the development of complications.

LOCAL

Lesions should be painted with 20% sulfonamide suspension, tincture of iodine or potassium permanganate 1:10,000 or a saturated solution of gentian violet.
Itching may be allayed by application of glycerin or nupercaine.

(Typical "take" with its corresponding Cross-Section)

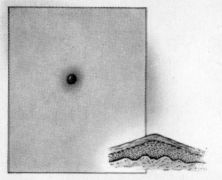

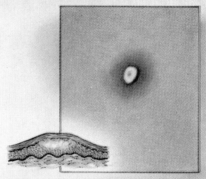

4th DAY — Papule appears round, red, flat and hard.

6th DAY — Vesicle appears like a pearl, becomes umbilicated and surrounded by red areola.

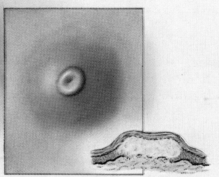

8th DAY — Enlarged vesicle becomes yellowish, fuller, umbilicated and the areola deeper, wider and edematous.

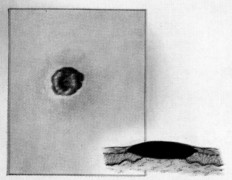

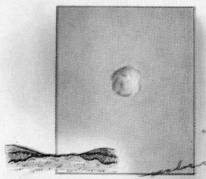

12th DAY — Brown wrinkled scab forms from the dried pustule.

24th DAY — Red scar turns white with typical pits or foveations.

REFERENCES:

COMBES, F. C., and BEHRMAN, H. T.: Eczema Vaccination, *New York State J. Med., 43:*2283, 1943.

EAGLES, F. H., and LEDINGHAM, J. C. G.: Vaccinia and the Paschen Body, *Lancet, 1:*823, 1932.

ELEY, R. C.: The Neurologic Complications of Vaccination, in Virus and Rickettsial Diseases, Cambridge, Harvard Univ. Press, 1940, p. 226.

ELLIS, F. A.: Eczema Vaccinatum: Its Relation to Generalized Vaccinia, *J.A.M.A., 104:*1891, 1935.

FLEXNER, S.: Postvaccinal Encephalitis and Allied Conditions, *J.A.M.A., 94:*305, 1930.

FOSTER, N. B.: A Puritan Practitioner, *Arch. Pediat., 39:*593, 1922.

GOODPASTURE, E. W., and BUDDINGH, G. J.: The Preparation of Antismallpox Vaccine by Culture of the Virus in the Chorioallantoic Membrane of Chick Embryos, and Its Use in Human Immunization, *Am. J. Hyg., 21:*319, 1935.

GORTER, E.: Postvaccinal Encephalitis, *J.A.M.A., 101:*1871, 1933.

GREEN, R. H., ANDERSON, T. F., and SINADEL, J. E.: Morphological Structure of the Virus of Vaccinia, *J. Exper. Med., 75:*651, 1942.

JENNER, E.: An Inquiry Into the Causes and Effects of the Variolae Vaccinae, A Disease Discovered in Some of the Western Counties of England Particularly Gloucestershire, and Known by the Name of Cowpox, London, Sampson Low, 1798.

RIVERS, T. M., WARD, S. M., and BAIRD, R. D.: Amount and Duration of Immunity Induced by Intradermal Inoculation of Cultured Vaccine Virus, *J. Exper. Med., 69:*857, 1939.

ROSS, R. A.: Generalized Vaccinia in Virus and Rickettsial Diseases, Cambridge, Harvard Univ. Press, 1940, p. 217.

XI

TETANUS

(LOCKJAW)

NATURE

Lockjaw is an acute intoxication of the central nervous system caused by Clostridium tetani.

It is characterized by stiffness of the skeletal muscles in any part of the body, particularly those of the jaw.

This is followed by painful trismus of the jaw, spasms and convulsions.

Symptoms develop after introduction of the bacilli as spores into a wound.

ETIOLOGY

The causative organism is usually present in cultivated ground, road dust and horse manure.

The bacillus is anaerobic and forms spores extremely resistant to heating and drying.

The organism is found normally in the intestinal canal of many herbivera.

A child becomes infected through contamination of a punctured wound, especially by splinters, nails, bee stings, insect bites, burns or bed sores.

PATHOGENESIS

The bacillus multiplies at the site of infection producing virulent water-soluble toxin.

This has special affinity for the central nervous system reached through lymphatics and bloodstream.

It combines with nerve tissues giving symptoms of the disease.

Toxins free in circulating blood can be neutralized by antitoxin.

Excess antitoxin maintained in the blood neutralizes fresh toxin formed in the wound.

There are 2 forms of tetanus, the general and the local but the latter is rare in children.

SYMPTOMS

NEWBORNS

Incubation period is several hours or days following contamination of umbilicus.

Onset is marked by restlessness, difficulty in nursing and painful cry.

Masseters become contracted and the jaws are forced open with difficulty.

Eyes are closed, forehead wrinkled and lips parted.

Opisthotonos is characteristic, respiration irregular, swallowing impossible.

Fever is slight, except terminally.

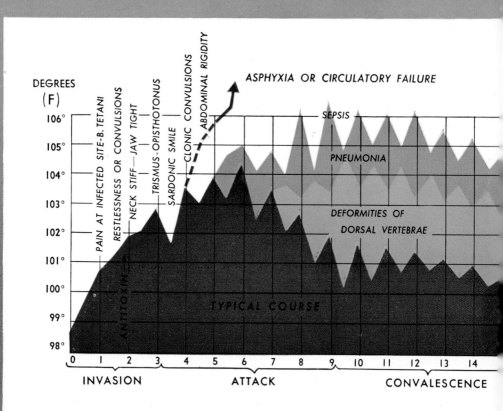

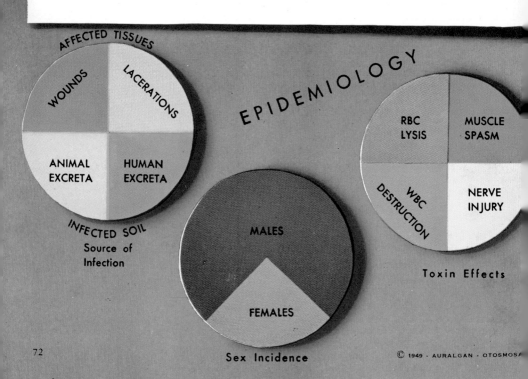

© 1949 · AURALGAN · OTOSMOSA

TETANUS — *continued*

CHILDREN AND ADULTS

Incubation period is 3 days to 3 weeks.
Headache, fever, chills, stiff neck precede difficulty in mastication.
Spasm of the musculature is typical.
Paroxysmal contraction of the muscles is recurrent.
Pain is intense in the spastic muscles.
Mind is clear.
Duration is 3 days in fatal cases.

PROGNOSIS

Mortality is between 30% and 50% in spite of therapy.
The disease is easy to prevent but difficult to treat.
Outlook is good in cases with long incubation period and local symptoms.
Outlook is bad with high fever, convulsions and persistent muscle spasms.

PROPHYLAXIS

PASSIVE IMMUNIZATION

Subcutaneous or intramuscular injection of 1,500 units of antitoxin must be preceded by skin tests for serum allergy.
This should be given with all cartilage wounds, puncture wounds, burns, lacerations and soil contamination.

ACTIVE IMMUNIZATION

Alum-precipitated toxin is given intramuscularly or subcutaneously.
The dose is 0.5 cc. for an infant and 1 cc. for a child, in 2 injections 1 month apart.

TREATMENT

GENERAL

The patient should be put into a dark room and protected from external stimuli.
Minimum handling is essential.
In severe cases of trismus, fluid is given by nasal catheter.
Sedatives are necessary to diminish the spasms.
Opiates must be avoided because of their depressing effect upon the respiratory centers.
Paraldehyde or avertin given rectally controls convulsive seizures.
Drinker respirator may become necessary.

SPECIFIC

Antitoxin neutralizes free toxin in circulation before it can attack susceptible nerve tissue.
It cannot affect toxin combined with nerve tissue.
After preliminary test for sensitivity to horse serum, inject tetanus antitoxin.

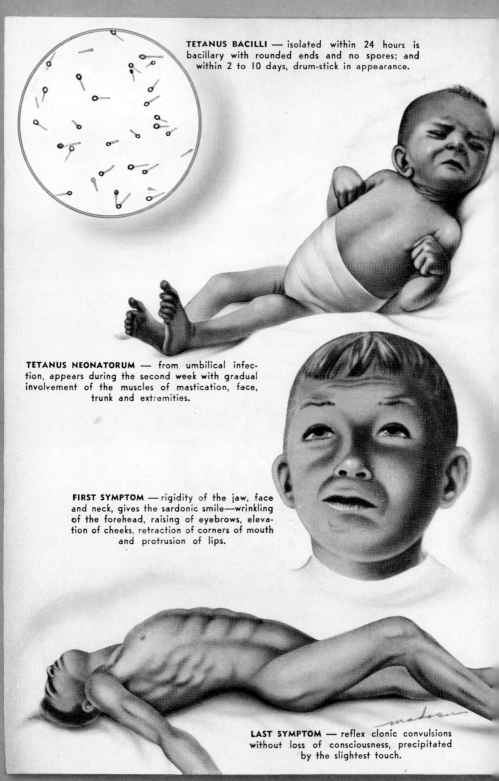

TETANUS BACILLI — isolated within 24 hours is bacillary with rounded ends and no spores; and within 2 to 10 days, drum-stick in appearance.

TETANUS NEONATORUM — from umbilical infection, appears during the second week with gradual involvement of the muscles of mastication, face, trunk and extremities.

FIRST SYMPTOM — rigidity of the jaw, face and neck, gives the sardonic smile—wrinkling of the forehead, raising of eyebrows, elevation of cheeks, retraction of corners of mouth and protrusion of lips.

LAST SYMPTOM — reflex clonic convulsions without loss of consciousness, precipitated by the slightest touch.

Inject 20,000 units around wound after local anesthesia. One hour later inject 60,000 units intramuscularly. Inject 40,000 units intravenously in 500 cc. saline giving epinephrine (1:1000) subcutaneously. Repeat 20,000 units intravenously 3 hours later. Give prophylactic dose for four doses q. 4 days to maintain serum desensitization.

Intrathecal antitoxin may be beneficial, 15,000-20,000 units given under anesthesia if necessary.

Penicillin in massive doses is effective but sulfonamides are valueless.

Infiltrate tissues around wound with 10,000 units serum one hour before excision.

REFERENCES:

VENER, H. I., BOWER, A. G., and McKILLOP, J. E.: Clinical Tetanus: A Study of 131 Cases, *California and West. Med., 39:*309, November, 1933.

COLE, L.: The Prognosis of Tetanus, *Lancet, 1:*164, Jan. 27, 1940.

FIROR, W. M., LAMONT, A., and SHUMACHER, H. B.: Cause of Death in Tetanus, *Ann. Surg., 111:*246, 1940.

GLENN, FRANK: Tetanus in the Battle of Manila, *Ann. Surg.,* 1946.

HUNTINGTON, R. W., JR., THOMPSON, W. R., and GORDON, H. H.: Treatment of Tetanus with Antitoxin: Analysis of Outcome in 642 Cases, *Ann. Surg., 195:* 93, January, 1937.

VENER, H. I.: Tetanus: Treatment, *California and West. Med., 48:*1, 1938.

VARNEY, P. L.: The Prophylaxis and Therapy of Tetanus, *Washington Univ. M. Alumni Quart., 3:*17, October, 1939.

XII

TYPHOID FEVER

NATURE

Enteric fever is an acute generalized infection caused by the Bacillus typhosus.
It is characterized clinically by high fever, slow pulse, rose-colored eruption,
abdominal distention and tenderness, and splenic enlargement.

It is characterized pathologically by hyperplasia and ulceration of Peyer's
patches and solitary lymph follicles of the intestinal tract, and swelling of
the mesenteric lymph nodes and spleen.

ETIOLOGY

The child may be infected by water, milk, dairy products, ice, salads, shell-
fish, flies or by direct contact with a typhoid carrier.

About 5% of those who have recovered from the disease continue to ex-
crete bacilli for months or years.

The incidence is greatest in the autumn and occasionally in any season.

It is a disease of youth and may even affect the newborn infant or fetus in
utero.

The infrequency of infantile typhoid is due to limited opportunity of contact
with the organism rather than to immunity.

The incubation period is 10 to 15 days.

PATHOLOGY

During the first 3 days typhoid fever is a blood infection, hence septicemia.
The organism may be recovered from both the blood and the urine at this
time.

Thereafter, the infection localizes in the lymphoid tissues of the bowel
causing hyperplasia and ulceration of Peyer's patches and swelling of the
mesenteric glands and of the spleen.

Cloudy swelling develops throughout all the organs.

There may be peripheral neuritis or encephalitis from these toxins.

Peyer's patches slough and separate leaving ulcers to perforate.

SYMPTOMS

FIRST WEEK

Chills at the onset accompany grippe-like symptoms.

Frontal or bitemporal headache and generalized aching.

Epistaxis is an early and persisting manifestation.

Nausea, vomiting, meteorism and constipation alternating with diarrhea.

Flushed face with dull, apathetic expression.

"Glassy" eyes, and hot, dry skin and mouth.

Coated tongue, white or brownish with reddened tip and edges.

Fever increasing daily in a step-like manner to 104° or 105° F.

CLINICAL COURSE OF TYPHOID FEVER

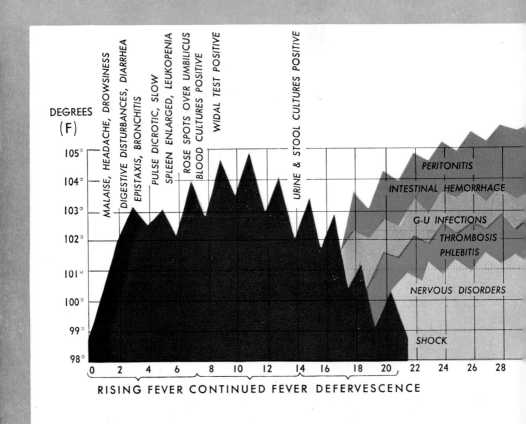

DEGREES (F)

MALAISE, HEADACHE, DROWSINESS

DIGESTIVE DISTURBANCES, DIARRHEA

EPISTAXIS, BRONCHITIS

PULSE DICROTIC, SLOW

SPLEEN ENLARGED, LEUKOPENIA

ROSE SPOTS OVER UMBILICUS

BLOOD CULTURES POSITIVE

WIDAL TEST POSITIVE

URINE & STOOL CULTURES POSITIVE

- 105°
- 104°
- 103°
- 102°
- 101°
- 100°
- 99°
- 98°

PERITONITIS

INTESTINAL HEMORRHAGE

G-U INFECTIONS

THROMBOSIS

PHLEBITIS

NERVOUS DISORDERS

SHOCK

0 2 4 6 8 10 12 14 16 18 20 22 24 26 28

RISING FEVER CONTINUED FEVER DEFERVESCENCE

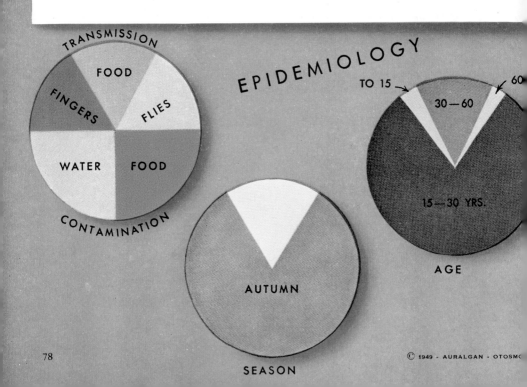

TRANSMISSION

FOOD

FINGERS

FLIES

WATER

FOOD

CONTAMINATION

EPIDEMIOLOGY

TO 15

30 — 60

60

15 — 30 YRS.

AGE

AUTUMN

SEASON

TYPHOID FEVER — *continued*

SECOND WEEK

Stupor and often muttering delirium with twitching of the muscles.
High fever, but slow, regular, full, dicrotic pulse.
Rose-colored rash, mainly on the abdomen but also on the chest and back. Successive crops of 2 or 3 days' duration of 1 to 20 round, pale pink, slightly elevated areas from 2 to 4 mm. in diameter fade momentarily on pressure.
Soft enlargement of the spleen rarely extends over 3 cm. below costal border.
Abdominal distention, tenderness and tympanites.
Constipation or diarrhea, often with incontinence of feces and urine.

THIRD WEEK

Greater remissions of the fever with a tendency to decline.
Smaller and less dicrotic pulse.
Gradual diminution of systemic manifestations.
Disappearance of the rash with a residual brownish stain.
Intestinal hemorrhage follows perforation of the intestine.

FOURTH WEEK

Gradual decline of the fever with greater remissions.
Gradual amelioration or disappearance of symptoms.

COMPLICATIONS

INTESTINAL

Gross hemorrhage and perforation due to erosion of an ulcer are rare.
Subnormal temperature, abdominal pain, vomiting, peritonitis and leukocytosis are indications for prompt surgical intervention.

HEPATIC

Jaundice from hepatitis may develop.
Persistent infection of the gallbladder is responsible for the carrier state and eventual cholelithiasis.

RESPIRATORY

The typhoid bacillus may be recovered from the sputum.
Otitis media, bronchitis and pneumonia occur in severe cases.

NERVOUS

The mental picture varies from delirium to stupor, due to toxicity.
Serous meningitis enables recovery of typhoid bacillus from the spinal fluid.
Psychoses from manic-depressive to melancholia disappear during convalescence.

SKIN

Furunculosis, bed sores and septicemia originate from skin infections.

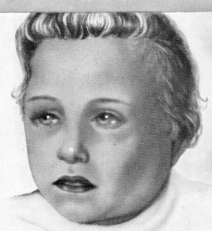

2nd WEEK — Parotitis due to lack of oral hygiene.

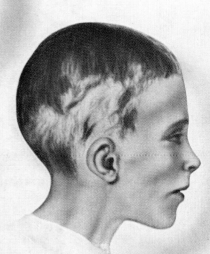

5th WEEK — Alopecia at the temple extending backwards elliptically.

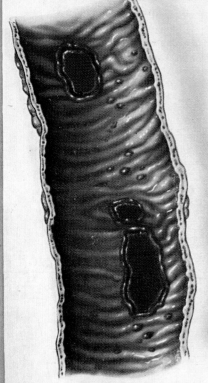

3rd WEEK — Intestinal hemorrhage and rarely perforation from erosion of blood vessels in ulcerated small intestine and necrosis of Peyer's patches.

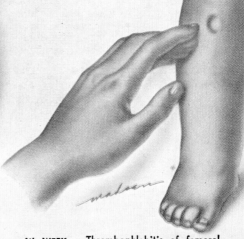

4th WEEK — Thrombophlebitis of femoral vein, pitting on pressure indicating lymph stasis and edema of the leg.

TYPHOID FEVER — *continued*

DIAGNOSIS

BLOOD

The leukocyte count is increased during the first few days but decreased thereafter until some complications develop. Lymphocytes are increased. Blood cultures are positive during the first week in 85% of the cases. Widal test is positive after the first week but a rising titer is diagnostic.

EXCRETA

Positive cultures from the urine and stools may be obtained throughout the disease.

PREVENTION

Vaccination with pure typhoid vaccine subcutaneously is effective for 3 years. One billion organisms per cc. is given in 3 weekly doses of 0.5, 1 and 1 cc., respectively, to children over 6 years of age and half this dose to infants. Revaccinations require only a single dose of 0.1 cc. given intradermally. Intracutaneous immunization with 0.1, 0.15 and 0.2 cc. combined vaccine eliminates reactions.

All exposed individuals should receive prophylactic inoculations.

Carriers may be given streptomycin, sulfonamide or iodophthalein.

TREATMENT

GENERAL

Bed rest is essential until the fever subsides.
Good nursing is of utmost importance.
Mouth hygiene prevents ulcer formation.
An air cushion prevents bed sores.
Excreta should be disinfected with 1:20 phenol.

SPECIFIC

Streptomycin, oral and parenteral, 1 million units daily for 14 days.
Sulfathalidine 3 gms. daily in divided doses and sulfapyridine in bacilluria.

NUTRITIONAL

A high caloric diet low in roughage offered in small amounts at frequent intervals, maintains strength and shortens convalescence.
Vitamin supplements prevent bleeding gums, nervous and mental symptoms.
Easily assimilable carbohydrates should be offered in fruit juices.
In dehydration, dextrose and saline should be given parenterally.

DRUGS

Antipyretic drugs depress the heart, hence tepid sponging is preferable.
Abdominal distention is combatted by turpentine stoops, rectal tube or enemata and administration of small doses of pitressin.
Diarrhea is treated by paregoric if bananas, apples and lactic acid milk are ineffective.

DIAGNOSTIC FEATURES OF TYPHOID FEVER

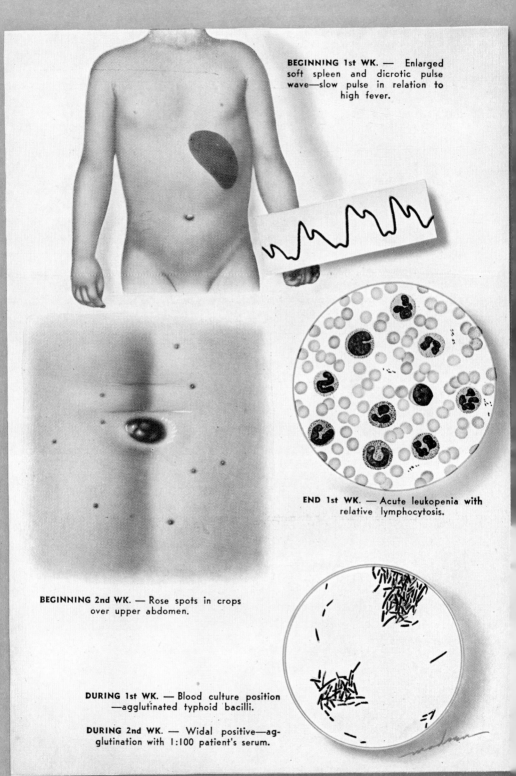

BEGINNING 1st WK. — Enlarged soft spleen and dicrotic pulse wave—slow pulse in relation to high fever.

END 1st WK. — Acute leukopenia with relative lymphocytosis.

BEGINNING 2nd WK. — Rose spots in crops over upper abdomen.

DURING 1st WK. — Blood culture position —agglutinated typhoid bacilli.

DURING 2nd WK. — Widal positive—ag- glutination with 1:100 patient's serum.

Hemorrhage requires morphine, an ice bag over the abdomen and a transfusion if necessary.

The blood must be carefully matched for hemolysis and agglutination.

SERUM

Antityphoid serum containing antibodies to the so-called O, H, Vi antigens may be effective in toxic cases if given early in the attack.

REFERENCES:

ANDERSON, G. W., HAMBLEN, A. D., and SMITH, H. M.: Typhoid Carriers; Study of Their Disease Producing Potentialities Over Series of Years as Indicated by Study of Cases, *Am. J. Pub. Health, 26:*396, April, 1936.

ELIOT, C. P.: The Vi Agglutination Test as Aid in Detection of Chronic Typhoid Carriers, *Am. J. Hyg. Sect. B, 31:*8, January, 1940.

FELIX, A.: Detection of Chronic Typhoid Carriers by Agglutination Tests, *Lancet, 2:*738, Sept. 24, 1938.

GRASSET, E.: Concentrated Anti-typhoid Serum as Specific in Treatment of Typhoid Fevers, *J. M. A. South Africa, 4:*380, July 12, 1930.

LEWIN, W.: Typhoid Fever on the Witwatersrand, *The South African Institute for Medical Research No. 41, 7:* Johannesburg, 1938.

McSWEENEY, C. J.: Serum Treatment of Typhoid Fever, *Brit. M. J., 2:*1118, Dec. 4, 1937.

REIMANN *et al*: Streptomycin for Typhoid, *J.A.M.A., 128:*175, 1945.

SILER, *et al.*: Duration of Immunity Conferred by Typhoid Vaccine, *Am. J. Pub. Health, 29:*75, 1939.

YU, H.: Further Studies on Serum Treatment of Typhoid Fever, *Chinese M. J., 56:* 29, July, 1939. Cited in *Bull. Hyg., 14:*805, November, 1939.

IMMUNIZATION SCHEDULE IN INFANCY AND EARLY CHILDHOOD

AGE	DISEASE	IMMUNIZING AGENT	ADMINISTRATION AND DOSAGE
3 months 4 months 5 months	Smallpox	Smallpox Vaccine	Apply contents of one capillary tube of smallpox vaccine by multiple puncture at any time between 3 and 6 months.
6 months	Whooping Cough Diphtheria and Tetanus	Diphtheria Tetanus Pertussis combined Each cc. contains 30 billion phase 1 H. pertussis organisms and one human immunizing dose each of diphtheria and tetanus toxoids.	Three subcutaneous injections of 1 cc. each at monthly intervals. First injection—1 cc. in left arm or buttock.
7 months	Whooping Cough Diphtheria and Tetanus	Same as above	Second injection—1 cc. in right arm or buttock.
8 months	Whooping Cough Diphtheria and Tetanus	Same as above	Third injection—1 cc. in left arm or buttock.
12-24 months	Scarlet Fever	Scarlet Fever Streptococcus Toxin Immunization is optional	Five injections of 650; 2,500; 10,000; 30,000 and 100,000 to 120,000 skin test doses subcutaneously at weekly intervals.

BOOSTER DOSES AND REIMMUNIZATION

AGE	DISEASE	IMMUNIZING AGENT	ADMINISTRATION AND DOSAGE
12-18 months	Whooping Cough Tetanus and Diphtheria	Same as above	1 cc. administered subcutaneously or intramuscularly.
5 years or when starting school or kindergarten	Whooping Cough Tetanus and Diphtheria	Same as above	A booster dose of 1 cc. administered deep subcutaneously or intramuscularly.
5 years or when starting school or kindergarten	Smallpox	Smallpox Vaccine	Apply one capillary tube by multiple puncture.

PARENTERAL THERAPY IN
SEVERE INFECTIONS

Dehydration without electrolyte imbalance

Infuse intravenously 5% dextrose in physiological saline.
Inject by clysis 5% dextrose in water, $2\frac{1}{2}$% dextrose and $2\frac{1}{2}$% saline or physiological saline.

Dehydration with metabolic acidosis

Infuse intravenously 10% dextrose containing one part 1/6 molar lactate or $NaHCO_3$, and two parts saline.
Inject by clysis 1/6 molar lactate solution.

Dehydration with metabolic alkalosis

Infuse intravenously 5% dextrose in saline (12 cc./min.).
Follow with 10% dextrose in saline 6 cc./min.

Dehydration with shock

Whole blood and plasma transfusions after fluid administration.

Daily Maintenance Requirements

	Water cc.	NaCl Gm.	Dextrose Gm./Kg. For Basic Caloric Needs	Amino Acids Gm./Kg. body weight
Infant	330-1000	1	15	1.5
Child	1000-1800	3	7	0.6
Adult	1800-2500	6	6	0.6

SULFONAMIDE THERAPY

PRECAUTIONS

Determine previous allergic history, including sulfonamide reactions.

Begin bacterial determinations before therapy.

Urinary output must be 1200-1500 cc. per day.

Normal renal function is a requisite for full dosage.

Choice of Drugs

Strep. Hemolyticus ....SD - SM - ST
Staphylococci ....ST - SD - SM
Pneumococci ....SD - SM - ST
Meningococci ....SD - SM - ST
Gonococci ....SD - SM - ST
Influenzal Bacillus ....SD - SM - ST
Friedländer's Bac. ....ST - SD - SM
Colon Bacillus ....ST - SD - SM

SD = Sulfadiazine   SM = Sulfamerazine   ST = Sulfathiazole

Maintenance Dose

Route	Sulfa	Initial Dose	Maintenance
Oral	S-thiazole	4 Gm.	1.0 Gm. q. 4h.
	S-diazine	4 Gm.	1.0 Gm. q. 4h.
	S-pyrazine	4 Gm.	1.0 Gm. q. 4h.
	S-merazine	4 Gm.	1.0 Gm. q. 6h.
Parenteral	S-thiazole	5 Gm. Intrav.	Orally as above
and Oral	S-diazine	5 Gm. "	" " "
	S-pyrazine	5 Gm. "	" " "
	S-merazine	5 Gm. "	" " "
Parenteral	S-thiazole	5 Gm. "	3 Gm. q. 12h.
	S-diazine	5 Gm. "	3 Gm. q. 12h.
	S-pyrazine	5 Gm. "	3 Gm. q. 12h.
	S-merazine	5 Gm. "	2 Gm. q. 12h.

Administration

Parenteral therapy. First dose in overwhelming injection, severe pneumonia or meningitis.

Vomiting, delirium or coma.

Insufficient blood level after oral dosage.

Toxicity

Renal complications: oliguria, anuria, gross hematuria.

Stop the drug immediately and determine N.P.N. and sulfonamide blood level.

1,500 cc. of saline intravenously with fluid intake of 4,000 cc. or more per 24 hours.

10 Gm. Sod. Bicarbonate orally, and 5 Gm. q. 2h. depending on urinary pH.

Bilateral ureteral lavage indicated if anuria or oliguria is present several hours without improvement.

Resume therapy with another sulfonamide only after free urinary flow is established and N.P.N. and urinary sediment have returned to normal. Penicillin may be used in the interim.

In acute hemolytic anemia, stop the sulfa and give large amounts of fluid, bicarbonate and blood.

In leukopenia, stop the sulfa, use penicillin, inject liver extract, pentonucleolide, pyridoxine or folic acid.

With rash and fever, stop the sulfa or change to penicillin.

With nausea and vomiting, do not stop the drug unless vomiting serious.

PENICILLIN THERAPY

Susceptible Organisms: Effective against Gram positive cocci and bacilli, Neisseria and spirochetes.

Doubtful against fungi; no effect against most Gram negative bacilli.

Order of Susceptibility: Gonococci, Streptococci, Pneumococci, Strep. Viridans, Meningococci, Staphylococci, Spirochetes, Clostridia, occasional strains of Gram negative bacilli.

Species Response: Staphylococci: susceptible with occasional resistant strains.

Streptococci: hemolytic responds best; resistant strains in anaerobic groups.

Pneumococci: resistance rare.

Neisseria: meningococcus responds better to sulfadiazine; gonococcus very susceptible.

Anthrax: responds well.

Clostridia: response with early antitoxin and surgery in gas gangrene.

C. diphtheriae: questionable clinically.

Treponemata: good when combined with arsenicals.

Rat bite fever organisms: good response.

Vincent's organisms: good response.

Actinomyces: irregular results.

CLINICAL COURSES OF INFECTIOUS DISEASES

DISEASE	·INCUBATION PERIOD	DURATION	QUARANTINE
Chicken pox	14-21 days	1-3 weeks	Until all crusts are off
Diphtheria	2-7 days	3 weeks	2 neg. throat cultures 10 days after onset
Dysentery, bacillary	1-4 days	3 weeks	3 weeks
Erysipelas	½-3 days	1-4 weeks	None
Erythema infectiosum	6-14 days	3-20 days	5 days after rash
Exanthem subitum	7-15 days	5-7 days	2 weeks
Fourth Disease	1-12 days	2-7 days	25 days after rash
Measles	7-18 days	2 weeks	5 days after rash disappears
Meningococcus Meningitis	2-4 days	3 weeks (may have relapse)	21 days
Pertussis	5-21 days	3-6 weeks	28 days
Poliomyelitis	3-20 days	3 weeks	21 days
Rocky Mountain Spotted and typhus fever	2-21 days	2-4 weeks	28 days
Rubella	5-21 days	4-8 days	5 days after rash
Scarlet fever	1-7 days	2-3 weeks	21 days if no ear or lymph node discharge
Smallpox	10-14 days	4-5 weeks	28 days or until the scabs disappear
Typhoid-para-typhoid fever	6-25 days	3-4 weeks	Until 2 successive stool cultures are negative
Vaccinia	3-6 days	10-15 days	None